Evidence-based Clinical Chinese Medicine

Volume 14

# Unipolar Depression

## Evidence-based Clinical Chinese Medicine

Co Editors-in-Chief

## Charlie Changli Xue
RMIT University, Australia

## Chuanjian Lu
Guangdong Provincial Hospital of Chinese Medicine, China

## Volume 14
# Unipolar Depression

Lead Authors

## Yuan Ming Di
RMIT University, Australia

## Lingling Yang
Guangdong Provincial Hospital of Chinese Medicine, China

## World Scientific

NEW JERSEY · LONDON · SINGAPORE · BEIJING · SHANGHAI · HONG KONG · TAIPEI · CHENNAI · TOKYO

*Published by*

World Scientific Publishing Co. Pte. Ltd.

5 Toh Tuck Link, Singapore 596224

*USA office:* 27 Warren Street, Suite 401-402, Hackensack, NJ 07601

*UK office:* 57 Shelton Street, Covent Garden, London WC2H 9HE

**Library of Congress Cataloging-in-Publication Data**
Names: Xue, Charlie Changli, author. | Lu, Chuan-jian, 1964–   author.
Title: Evidence-based clinical Chinese medicine / Charlie Changli Xue, Chuanjian Lu.
Description: New Jersey : World Scientific, 2016. | Includes bibliographical references and index.
Identifiers: LCCN 2015030389| ISBN 9789814723084 (v. 1 : hardcover : alk. paper) |
    ISBN 9789814723091 (v. 1 : paperback : alk. paper) |
    ISBN 9789814723121 (v. 2 : hardcover : alk. paper) |
    ISBN 9789814723138 (v. 2 : paperback : alk. paper) |
    ISBN 9789814759045 (v. 3 : hardcover : alk. paper) |
    ISBN 9789814759052 (v. 3 : paperback : alk. paper)
Subjects: | MESH: Medicine, Chinese Traditional--methods. | Clinical Medicine--methods. |
    Evidence-Based Medicine--methods. | Psoriasis. | Pulmonary Disease, Chronic Obstructive.
Classification: LCC RC81 | NLM WB 55.C4 | DDC 616--dc23
LC record available at http://lccn.loc.gov/2015030389

**Volume 14: Unipolar Depression**
ISBN  978-981-120-597-2 (hardcover)
ISBN  978-981-120-598-9 (ebook for institutions)
ISBN  978-981-120-599-6 (ebook for individuals)

**British Library Cataloguing-in-Publication Data**
A catalogue record for this book is available from the British Library.

For any available supplementary material, please visit
https://www.worldscientific.com/worldscibooks/10.1142/11435#t=suppl

# Disclaimer

The information in this monograph is based on systematic analyses of the best available evidence for Chinese medicine interventions both historical and contemporary. Every effort has been made to ensure accuracy and completeness of the data of this publication. This book is intended for clinicians, researchers and educators. The practice of evidence-based medicine consists of consideration of the best available evidence, practitioners' clinical experience and judgment, and patients' preference. Not all interventions are acceptable in all countries. It is important to note that some of the substances mentioned in this book may no longer be in use, may be toxic, or be prohibited or restricted under the provisions of the Convention on International Trade in Endangered Species of Wild Fauna and Flora (CITES). Practitioners, researchers and educators are advised to comply with the relevant regulations in their country and with the restrictions on the trade in species included in CITES appendices I, II and III. This book is not intended as a guide for self-medication. Patients should seek professional advice from qualified Chinese medicine practitioners.

# Foreword

Since the late 20th century, Chinese medicine, including acupuncture and herbal medicine, has been increasingly used throughout the world. The parallel development and spread of evidence-based medicine has provided challenges and opportunities for Chinese medicine. The opportunities have been evidence-based medicine's emphasis on the effective use of the best available clinical evidence, incorporating the clinicians' clinical experience, subject to patients' preference. Such practices have a patient focus which reflects the historical nature of Chinese medicine practice. However, the challenges are also significant due to the fact that, despite the long-term development and very rich literature accumulated over 2,000 years, there is an overall lack of high level clinical evidence for many of the interventions used in Chinese medicine.

To address this knowledge gap, we need to generate clinical evidence through high quality clinical studies and to evaluate evidence to enable effective use of such available evidence to promote evidence-based Chinese medicine practice.

Modern Chinese medicine is rooted in its classical literature and the legacies of ancient doctors, grounded in the practice of expert clinicians and increasingly informed by clinical and experimental research efforts. In recognition of the unique features of Chinese medicine, for each of the conditions in this series a "Whole Evidence" approach is used to provide a synthesis of different types and levels of evidence to enable practitioners to make clinical decisions informed by the current best evidence.

There are four main components of this "Whole Evidence" approach. Firstly, we present the current approaches to the diagnosis, differentiation and treatment of each condition based on expert consensus in published textbooks and clinical guidelines. This provides an overview of how the condition is currently managed. The second section provides an analysis of the condition in historical context based on systematic searches of the *Zhong Hua Yi Dian* which includes the full texts of more than 1,000 classical medical books. These analyses provide objective views on how the condition has been treated over two millennia, reveal continuities and discontinuities between traditional and modern practice, and suggest avenues for future research.

The third component is the assessment of evidence derived from modern clinical studies of Chinese medicine interventions. The methods established by the *Cochrane Collaboration* are used as the basis for conducting systematic reviews and undertaking meta-analyses of outcome data for randomised controlled trials (RCTs). In addition, the clinical relevance of meta-analysis data is enhanced by examining the herbal formulae, individual herbs and acupuncture treatments that were assessed in the RCTs and the evidence base is broadened by the inclusion of data from controlled clinical trials and non-controlled studies. The fourth component is to determine how the herbal medicine interventions may achieve the effects indicated by the clinical trials. Thus for each of the most frequently used herbs we provide reviews of their effects in pre-clinical models and their likely mechanisms of action.

For each condition, this "Whole Evidence" approach links clinical expertise, historical precedent, clinical research data and experimental research to provide the reader with assessments of the current state of the evidence of efficacy and safety for Chinese medicine interventions using herbal medicines, acupuncture and moxibustion and other healthcare practices such as *tai chi*.

Since these books are available in Chinese and English, they can benefit patients, practitioners and educators internationally and enable practitioners to make clinical decisions informed by the current best evidence.

These publications represent a major milestone in Chinese medicine development and make a significant contribution to the evidence-based Chinese medicine development globally.

**Co-Editors-in-Chief**

Professor Charlie Changli Xue, RMIT University, Australia

Professor Chuanjian Lu, Guangdong Provincial Hospital of Chinese Medicine, China

# Purpose of the Monograph

This book is intended for clinicians, researchers and educators. It can be used to inform tertiary education and clinical practice by providing systematic, multi-dimensional assessments of the best available evidence for using Chinese medicine to manage each common clinical condition.

## How to Use this Monograph

### Some Definitions

A glossary is included, containing terms and definitions which frequently appear in the book. It also describes the definitions of statistical tests, methodological terms, evaluation tools and interventions. For example, in this book, Integrative Medicine refers to the combined use of a Chinese medicine treatment with conventional medical management, and Combination Therapies refers to two or more Chinese medicines from different therapy groups (Chinese herbal medicine, acupuncture or other Chinese medicine therapies) administered together. Terminology used throughout the monograph is based on the World Health Organisation's *Standard Terminologies on Traditional Medicine in the Western Pacific Region* (2007) where possible or from the cited reference.

### Data Analysis and Interpretation of Results

In order to synthesise the clinical evidence, a range of statistical analysis approaches are used. In general, the effect size for dichotomous data is reported as a risk ratio (RR) with 95% confidence intervals (CI), and for continuous data, they are reported as mean difference (MD) with 95% CI. Statistically significant effects are indicated with an asterisk*. Readers should note that statistical significance does not necessarily correspond with a clinically important effect. Interpretation of results should take into consideration of the clinical significance, quality of studies (expressed as high, low or unclear risk of bias in this book) and heterogeneity amongst the studies. Tests for heterogeneity are conducted using the $I^2$ statistic. An $I^2$ score greater than 50% may indicate substantial heterogeneity.

## Use of Evidence in Practice

The Grading of Recommendations Assessment, Development and Evaluation (GRADE) approach was used to summarise the quality of evidence and results of the strength of evidence for critical and important comparisons and outcomes. Due to the diverse nature of Chinese medicine practice, treatment recommendations are not included with the summary of findings tables. Therefore readers will need to interpret the evidence with reference to the local practice environment.

## Limitations

Readers should note some of the methodological limitations on classical literature and clinical evidence.

- Search terms used to search the *Zhong Hua Yi Dian* database may not include all terms that have been used for the condition, which may alter the findings.
- Chinese language has changed over time. Citations have been interpreted for analysis, and such interpretations may be subject to disagreement.
- Chinese medicine theory has evolved over time. As such, concepts described in classical Chinese medical literature may no longer be found in contemporary works.

- Symptoms described in citations may be common to many conditions, and a judgment was required to determine the likelihood of the citation being related to the condition. This may have introduced some bias due to the subjective nature of the judgment.
- The vast majority of the clinical evidence for Chinese medicine treatments has come from China. The applicability of the findings to other populations and other countries requires further assessment.
- Many studies included participants with varying disease severity. Where possible, subgroup analyses were undertaken to examine the effects in different sub-populations. As this was not always possible, the findings may be limited to the population included, and not to sub-populations.
- The potential risk of bias found in many included studies suggested methodological limitations. The findings for GRADE assessments based on studies of very low to moderate quality evidence should be interpreted accordingly.
- Nine major English and Chinese language databases were searched to identify clinical studies, in addition to clinical trial registers. Other studies may exist which were not identified through searches, and which may alter the findings.
- The calculation of frequency of herbal formula use was based on formula names only. It is possible that studies evaluated herbal treatments with the same or similar herb ingredients, but which were given different formula names. Due to the complexity of herbal formulas, it was considered not appropriate to make a judgment as to the similarity of formulas for analysis. As such, the frequency of formulas reported in Chapter 5 may be underestimated.
- The most frequently utilised herbs which may have contributed to the treatment effect have been described in Chapter 5. These herbs may provide leads for further exploration. Calculation of the herbs with potential effect is based on frequency of formulae reported in the studies, and doesn't take into consideration the clinical implications and functions of every herb in a formula.

# Authors and Contributors

CO-EDITORS-IN-CHIEF

Prof. Charlie Changli Xue (*RMIT University, Australia*)
Prof. Chuanjian Lu (*Guangdong Provincial Hospital of Chinese Medicine, China*)

CO-DEPUTY EDITORS-IN-CHIEF

Assoc. Prof. Anthony Lin Zhang (*RMIT University, Australia*)
Dr. Brian H May (*RMIT University, Australia*)
Prof. Xinfeng Guo (*Guangdong Provincial Hospital of Chinese Medicine, China*)
Prof. Zehuai Wen (*Guangdong Provincial Hospital of Chinese Medicine, China*)

LEAD AUTHORS

Dr. Yuan Ming Di (*RMIT University, Australia*)
Dr. Lingling Yang (*Guangdong Provincial Hospital of Chinese Medicine, China*)

CO-AUTHORS

*RMIT University (Australia):*
Dr. Johannah Shergis
Assoc. Prof. Anthony Lin Zhang
Prof. Charlie Changli Xue

*Guangdong Provincial Hospital of Chinese Medicine (China):*
Prof. Yan Li
Prof. Chuanjian Lu
Prof. Xinfeng Guo

# Member of Advisory Committee and Panel

## CO-CHAIRS OF PROJECT PLANNING COMMITTEE

Prof. Dacan Chen (*Guangdong Provincial Hospital of Chinese Medicine, China*)

Prof. Peter J Coloe (*RMIT University, Australia*)

Prof. Yubo Lyu (*Guangdong Provincial Hospital of Chinese Medicine, China*)

## CENTRE ADVISORY COMMITTEE (ALPHABETICAL ORDER)

Prof. Keji Chen (*The Chinese Academy of Sciences, China*)

Prof. Aiping Lu (*Hong Kong Baptist University, China*)

Prof. Caroline Smith (*University of Western Sydney, Australia*)

Prof. David F Story (*RMIT University, Australia*)

## METHODOLOGY EXPERT ADVISORY PANEL (ALPHABETICAL ORDER)

Prof. Zhaoxiang Bian (*Hong Kong Baptist University, China*)

Prof. Lixing Lao (*The University of Hong Kong, China*)

The Late Prof. George Lewith (*University of Southampton, United Kingdom*)

Prof. Jianping Liu (*Beijing University of Chinese Medicine, China*)

Prof. Frank Thien (*Monash University, Australia*)

Prof. Jialiang Wang (*Sichuan University, China*)

## CONTENT EXPERT ADVISORY PANEL (ALPHABETICAL ORDER)

Prof. Yuping Ning (*Guangzhou Huiai Hospital/The Affiliated Brain Hospital of Guangzhou Medical University, China*)

Dr. Jerome Sarris (*Western Sydney University, Australia*)

Prof. Weikang Wu (*Sun Yat-sen University, China*)

# Professor Charlie Changli Xue, PhD

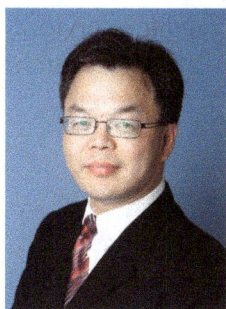

Professor Charlie Changli Xue holds a Bachelor of Medicine (majoring in Chinese Medicine) from Guangzhou University of Chinese Medicine, China (1987) and a PhD from RMIT University, Australia (2000). He has been an academic, researcher, regulator and practitioner for almost three decades. Professor Xue has made significant contributions to evidence-based educational development, clinical research, regulatory framework and policy development and provision of high quality clinical care to the community. Professor Xue is recognised internationally as an expert in evidence-based traditional medicine and integrative healthcare.

Professor Xue is the Inaugural National Chair of the Chinese Medicine Board of Australia appointed by the Australian Health Workforce Ministerial Council (in 2011), and he was reappointed for the second term in 2014. Since 2007, he has been a Member of the World Health Organization (WHO) Expert Advisory Panel for Traditional and Complementary Medicine, Geneva. Professor Xue is also Honorary Senior Principal Research Fellow at the Guangdong Provincial Academy of Chinese Medical Sciences, China.

At RMIT, Professor Xue is Executive Dean, School of Health and Biomedical Sciences. He is also Director, World Health Organization (WHO) Collaborating Centre for Traditional Medicine.

Between 1995 and 2010, Professor Xue was Discipline Head of Chinese Medicine at RMIT University. He leads the development of five successful undergraduate and postgraduate degree programs in

Chinese Medicine at RMIT University which is now a global leader in Chinese medicine education and research.

Professor Xue's research has been supported by over AU$15 million research grants including six project grants from the Australian Government's National Health & Medical Research Council (NHMRC) and two Australian Research Council (ARC) grants. He has contributed over 200 publications and has been frequently invited as keynote speaker for numerous national and international conferences. Professor Xue has contributed to over 300 media interviews on issues related to complementary medicine education, research, regulation and practice.

# Professor Chuanjian Lu, MD

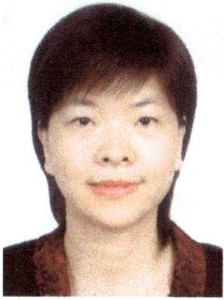

Professor Chuanjian Lu, Doctor of Medicine. She is the vice president of Guangdong Provincial Hospital of Chinese Medicine (Guangdong Provincial Academy of Chinese Medical Sciences, Second Clinical Medical College of Guangzhou University of Chinese Medicine). She is also the chair of the Guangdong Traditional Chinese Medicine (TCM) Standardization Technical Committee, and the vice-chair of the Immunity Specialty Committee of the World Federation of Chinese Medicine Societies (WFCMS).

Professor Lu has engaged in scientific research into TCM, clinical practice and teaching for some 25 years. Her research has been devoted to integrated traditional and Western medicine. She has edited and published 12 monographs and 120 academic research articles as first author and corresponding author with over 30 articles being included in SCI journals. She has received widespread recognition for her achievements with awards for "Excellent Teacher of South China", "National Outstanding Women TCM Doctor", and "National Outstanding Young Doctor of TCM". She also received "The Science and Technology Star of the Association of Chinese Medicine", the "National Excellent Science and Technology Workers of China Award" and the "Five-Continent Women's Scientific Awards of China Medical Women's Association".

Professor Lu has won the Award of Science and Technology Progress over 10 times from Guangdong Provincial Government, China Association of Chinese Medicine and Chinese Hospital Association.

# Acknowledgements

The authors and contributors would like to acknowledge the valuable contributions of the following people who assisted with database searches, data extraction, data screening, data assessment, translation of documents, editing, and/or administrative tasks: Dr. Jhodie Duncan, Zenan Fang, Chunyi Zhao, Jing Chen.

# Contents

| | |
|---|---|
| *Disclaimer* | v |
| *Foreword* | vii |
| *Purpose of the Monograph* | xi |
| *Authors and Contributors* | xv |
| *Member of Advisory Committee and Panel* | xvii |
| *Professor Charlie Changli Xue, PhD* | xix |
| *Professor Chuanjian Lu, MD* | xxi |
| *Acknowledgements* | xxiii |
| *List of Figures* | xxxv |
| *List of Tables* | xxxvii |

| | |
|---|---|
| **1. Introduction to Unipolar Depression** | **1** |
| Definition and Clinical Presentation of Unipolar Depression | 1 |
| Epidemiology | 2 |
| Burden | 2 |
| Risk Factors | 4 |
| Pathological Processes | 4 |
| Diagnosis | 6 |
| Management | 9 |
| Treatment Phases | 10 |
| Acute Phase Treatment | 10 |
| Continuation Phase Treatment | 11 |
| Maintenance Phase Treatment | 11 |
| Discontinuation of Treatment and Monitoring | 12 |
| Pharmacological Treatments | 12 |
| Non-pharmacological Treatments | 14 |
| Prevention | 15 |

Prognosis                                                      15
References                                                     16

**2. Unipolar Depression in Chinese Medicine**                **21**
Introduction                                                   21
Aetiology and Pathogenesis                                     22
Syndrome Differentiation and Treatments                        23
   Treatment Based on Syndrome Differentiation  24
   Liver *Qi* Stagnation                        25
   Liver *Qi* Stagnation and Phlegm Stagnation  25
   Liver *Qi* Stagnation and Spleen *Qi* Deficiency  26
   *Qi* Stagnation Transforming into Fire       27
   *Qi* Stagnation with Blood Stasis            27
   Liver-Gallbladder Damp-heat                  28
   *Yin* Deficiency with Fire                   29
   Deficiency of the Heart and Spleen           30
   Heart and Kidney *Yin* Deficiency            30
   Melancholy Disturbing the Mind               31
Acupuncture Therapies                                          31
   Acupuncture Treatment Based on Syndrome
    Differentiation                         32
Other Management Strategies                                    33
   Diet Therapy                                 33
References                                                     33

**3. Classical Chinese Medicine Literature**                  **35**
Introduction                                                   35
Search Terms                                                   36
Search Procedure and Data Coding                               36
Data Analysis Procedure                                        37
Search Results                                                 38
   Frequency of Treatment Citations by Dynasty  39
Definitions of the Condition and Aetiology                     40
Chinese Herbal Medicine                                        41
   Most Frequent Formulae in Depression Citations  41
   Most Frequent Herbs in Depression Citations  43

Herbal Wash                                                45
Combination Therapies                                      45
Acupuncture and related Therapies                          46
Discussion                                                 48
Classical Literature in Perspective                        49
References                                                 50

**4. Methods for Evaluating Clinical Evidence              53**
Introduction                                               53
Search Strategy                                            54
  Inclusion Criteria                                       56
  Exclusion Criteria                                       57
Outcomes                                                   57
  Hamilton Rating Scale for Depression                     57
  Montgomery–Asberg Depression Rating Scale                58
  Beck Depression Inventory                                58
  Zung Self-rating Depression Scale                        58
  Edinburgh Postnatal Depression Scale                     59
  Treatment Emergent Symptom Scale                         59
  Rating Scale for Side Effects — Asberg                   59
  World Health Organisation Quality of Life Scale
    Brief Version                                          59
Risk of Bias Assessment                                    60
Statistical Analyses                                       61
  Assessment Using Grading of Recommendations
    Assessment, Development and Evaluation                 62
References                                                 64

**5. Clinical Evidence for Chinese Herbal Medicine         67**
Introduction                                               67
Previous Systematic Reviews                                67
Identification of Clinical Studies                         70
Chinese Herbal Medicine Treatments                         72
Randomised Controlled Trials of Chinese Herbal Medicine    73
Risk of Bias                                               76
Results of Meta-analyses                                   76

Hamilton Rating Scale for Depression 77
Chinese Herbal Medicine vs. Placebo 77
Chinese Herbal Medicine vs. Antidepressants 77
Chinese Herbal Medical plus Antidepressants vs.
Antidepressants: Integrative Medicine 82
Chinese Herbal Medicine plus Antidepressants
and Psychotherapy vs. Antidepressants plus
Psychotherapy 86
Zung Self-rating Depression Scale 86
Chinese Herbal Medicine vs. Antidepressants 86
Chinese Herbal Medicine plus Antidepressants vs.
Antidepressants 87
Montgomery–Asberg Depression Scale 87
Chinese Herbal Medicine vs. Antidepressants 87
Chinese Herbal Medicine plus Antidepressants vs.
Antidepressants 87
Edinburgh Postnatal Depression Scale 87
Chinese Herbal Medicine vs. Placebo 88
Chinese Herbal Medicine vs. Antidepressants 88
Chinese Herbal Medicine plus Antidepressants vs.
Antidepressants 88
Chinese Herbal Medicine plus Psychotherapy vs.
Psychotherapy 88
Effective Rate 88
Chinese Herbal Medicine vs. Antidepressants 88
Chinese Herbal Medicine plus Antidepressants vs.
Antidepressants 89
Chinese Herbal Medicine plus Psychotherapy vs.
Psychotherapy 89
Assessment Using GRADE 89
Randomised Controlled Trial Evidence for Individual
Formulae 92
Xiao yao san/wan 逍遥散/丸 92
Hamilton Rating Scale for Depression 92
Treatment Emergent Symptom Scale 92
Adverse Events 92

Chai hu shu gan san 柴胡疏肝散 93

  Hamilton Rating Scale for Depression 93

  Adverse Events 93

Dan zhi xiao yao san 丹栀逍遥散 93

  Hamilton Rating Scale for Depression 93

  Self-rating Depression Scale 94

  Side Effect Rating Scales of Asberg 94

An shen ding zhi tang 安神定志汤 94

  Hamilton Rating Scale for Depression 94

  Treatment Emergent Symptom Scale 94

  Adverse Events 94

Bu shen shu gan hua yu tang 补肾疏肝化瘀汤 95

Jia wei xiao yao capsules 加味逍遥胶囊 95

  Hamilton Rating Scale for Depression 95

  Adverse Events 95

Frequently Reported Used Herbs in Meta-analyses
Showing Favourable Effect 95

Safety of Chinese Herbal Medicine in Randomised
Controlled Trials 97

  Treatment Emergent Symptom Scale 97

  Side Effect Rating Scales of Asberg 97

  Adverse Events 97

    Chinese Herbal Medicine vs. Placebo 99

    Chinese Herbal Medicine vs. Antidepressants 99

    Chinese Herbal Medicine plus Antidepressants vs.
Antidepressants 100

    Chinese Herbal Medicine plus Antidepressants and
Psychotherapy vs. Antidepressants and Psychotherapy 100

Controlled Clinical Trials of Chinese Herbal Medicine 101

  Hamilton Rating Scale for Depression 101

  Zung Self-rating Depression Scale 101

  Safety of Chinese Herbal Medicine in Controlled Clinical
Trials 102

Non-controlled Studies of Chinese Herbal Medicine 102

  Safety of Chinese Herbal Medicine in Non-controlled
Studies 102

Clinical Evidence for Commonly Used Chinese Herbal
   Medicine Treatments   103
Ban xia hou po tang 半夏厚朴汤   103
Gui pi tang 归脾汤   103
Yue ju wan 越鞠丸   104
Summary of Chinese Herbal Medicine Clinical Evidence   104
Chinese Herbal Medicine   105
Integrative Medicine   106
References   107

**6. Pharmacological Actions of Frequently Used Herbs**   **117**
Introduction   117
Methods   118
Experimental Studies on *chai hu*   118
Experimental Studies on *shao yao*   119
Experimental studies on *gan cao*   121
Experimental Studies on *yuan zhi*   122
Experimental Studies on *shi chang pu*   123
Experimental Studies on *zhi ke*   124
Experimental Studies on *di huang*   125
Experimental Studies on *dan shen*   125
Experimental Studies on *Xiao yao san*   126
Experimental Studies on *Chai hu shu gan san*   127
Summary of Pharmacological Actions   128
References   128

**7. Clinical Evidence for Acupuncture and Related
Therapies**   **133**
Introduction   133
Previous Systematic Reviews   134
Identification and Characteristics of Clinical Studies   135
Risk of Bias   137
Acupuncture   138
Randomised Controlled Trials of Acupuncture   138

Acupuncture vs. Antidepressants 138
   Hamilton Rating Scale for Depression 138
   World Health Organization Quality of Life
      Questionnaire 141
Acupuncture plus Antidepressants vs. Antidepressants 141
   Hamilton Rating Scale for Depression 141
   Montgomery–Asberg Depression Scale 143
   Zung Self-rating Depression Scale 143
   Relapse Rate 143
Controlled Clinical Trials of Acupuncture 143
Non-controlled Studies of Acupuncture 143
Safety of Acupuncture 144
Electroacupuncture 144
Randomised Controlled Trials of Electroacupuncture 145
Electroacupuncture vs. Sham Electroacupuncture 145
   Hamilton Rating Scale for Depression 145
   Zung Self-rating Depression Scale 145
Electroacupuncture vs. Antidepressants 145
   Hamilton Rating Scale for Depression 145
   Zung Self-rating Depression Scale 147
   World Health Organization Quality of Life
      Questionnaire 147
Electroacupuncture Plus Antidepressants vs.
   Antidepressants 147
   Hamilton Rating Scale for Depression 147
   Zung Self-rating Depression Scale 148
Electroacupuncture vs. Psychotherapy 148
Electroacupuncture plus Psychotherapy vs. Psychotherapy 148
Controlled Clinical Trials of Electroacupuncture 148
Non-controlled Studies of Electroacupuncture 148
Safety of Electroacupuncture 148
Acupuncture-related Therapies 149
Transcutaneous Electrical Nerve Stimulation 149
Laser Therapy 150

Frequently Reported Acupuncture Points in
  Meta-analyses Showing Favourable Effect 150
Assessment Using GRADE 150
Summary of Acupuncture and Related Therapies 153
References 154

**8. Clinical Evidence for Other Chinese Medicine Therapies 159**
Introduction 159
Previous Systematic Reviews 159
Identification of Clinical Studies 159
  Cupping Therapy 161
  Tuina 161
Summary of Other Chinese Medicine 161

**9. Clinical Evidence for Combination Therapies 163**
Introduction 163
Randomised Controlled Trials of Combination Therapies 163
Risk of Bias 165
Clinical Evidence for Combination Therapies from
  Randomised Controlled Trials 166
  Acupuncture plus Chinese Herbal Medicine vs.
    Antidepressants 166
  Acupuncture plus Chinese Herbal Medicine vs. Placebo 166
  Acupuncture plus *Tuina* vs. Antidepressants 168
  Acupuncture plus Moxibustion vs. Antidepressants 168
  Acupuncture plus Moxibustion plus Five-element
    Music Therapy vs. Antidepressants 168
  Acupuncture plus Cupping plus Psychotherapy
    vs. Psychotherapy 168
  Qigong, Tuina, and Taichi plus Antidepressants vs.
    Antidepressants 169
Controlled Clinical Trials of Combination Therapies 169
Non-controlled Studies of Combination Therapies 169
Summary of Combination Therapies 169

**10. Summary and Conclusions**                                    **171**
   Introduction                                                      171
   Chinese Medicine Syndrome Differentiation                        172
   Chinese Herbal Medicine                                          173
      Chinese Herbal Medicine Formulae in Key Clinical
         Guidelines and Textbooks, Classical Literature and
         Clinical Studies                                           175
   Acupuncture and Related Therapies                                178
   Other Chinese Medicine Therapies                                 180
   Limitations of Evidence                                          181
   Implications for Practice                                        183
   Implications for Research                                        184
   References                                                       185

**Glossary**                                                        **187**

**Index**                                                           **195**

# List of Figures

Figure 5.1.  Flow Chart of Study Selection Process: Chinese
             herbal medicine                                    71
Figure 7.1.  Flow Chart of Study Selection Process:
             Acupuncture and Related Therapies                 136
Figure 8.1.  Flow Chart of Study Selection Process: Other
             Chinese Medicine Therapies                        160
Figure 9.1.  Flow Chart of Study Selection Process:
             Combination Therapies                             164

# List of Tables

Table 1.1.  Treatment Phases of Depression                    10
Table 1.2.  Pharmacological Treatments for Depression         13
Table 2.1.  Summary of Chinese Herbal Medicines for
            Depression                                        24
Table 3.1.  Hit Frequency by Search Term                      38
Table 3.2.  Dynastic Distribution of Treatment Citations      40
Table 3.3.  Most Frequent Formulae in Depression Citations    42
Table 3.4.  Most Frequent Herbs in Depression Citations       44
Table 4.1.  Chinese Medicine Interventions Included
            in Clinical Evidence Evaluation                   54
Table 4.2.  Pre-specified Outcomes                            56
Table 5.1.  Frequently Reported Formulae in Randomised
            Controlled Trials                                 74
Table 5.2.  Frequently Reported Herbs in Randomised
            Controlled Trials                                 74
Table 5.3.  Risk of Bias of Randomised Controlled Trials      76
Table 5.4.  Chinese Herbal Medicine vs. Antidepressants:
            Hamilton Rating Scale for Depression              78
Table 5.5.  Chinese Herbal Medicine Plus Antidepressants
            vs. Antidepressants: Hamilton Rating Scale for
            Depression                                        83
Table 5.6.  GRADE: Chinese Herbal Medicine vs.
            Antidepressants                                   90
Table 5.7.  GRADE: Chinese Herbal Medicine Plus
            Antidepressants vs. Antidepressants               91
Table 5.8.  Frequently Reported Herbs in Meta-analyses
            Showing Favourable Effect                         96
Table 5.9.  Adverse Events                                    98

Table 7.1.   Risk of Bias of Randomised Controlled Trials            137
Table 7.2.   Acupuncture vs. Antidepressant: Hamilton
             Rating Scale for Depression                             139
Table 7.3.   Acupuncture Plus Antidepressants vs.
             Antidepressants: Hamilton Rating Scale for
             Depression                                              142
Table 7.4.   Electroacupuncture vs. Antidepressants:
             Hamilton Rating Scale for Depression                    146
Table 7.5.   GRADE: Acupuncture vs. Antidepressants                  151
Table 7.6.   GRADE: Acupuncture Plus Antidepressants vs.
             Antidepressants                                         152
Table 9.1.   Risk of Bias of Randomised Controlled Trials:
             Combination Therapies                                   165
Table 9.2.   Evidence for Combination Therapies from
             Randomised Controlled Trials                            167
Table 10.1. Summary of Chinese Herbal Medicine Formulae              176
Table 10.2. Summary of Acupuncture and Related Therapies             179
Table 10.3. Summary of Other Chinese Medicine Therapies              181

# 1

# Introduction to Unipolar Depression

## OVERVIEW

Unipolar depression, also known as major depressive disorder, is a mental disorder that is characterised by depressed mood and loss of interest in activities leading to impairment in daily life. Unipolar depression affects millions of people worldwide and its impact is ever increasing due to population growth and ageing. It may present as an isolated event, occur episodically or remain persistently. The causes are numerous and may include genetic predisposition, change in life circumstances, traumatic events or fluctuating hormones. Treatment often involves cognitive behavioural therapy and pharmacotherapy such as antidepressants. This chapter describes the definition, risk factors, epidemiological profile, pathological processes, diagnosis and treatment of unipolar depression.

## Definition and Clinical Presentation of Unipolar Depression

The term depression can refer to depressed mood state, depressive syndromes or a specific clinical condition, or a diagnosed mental disorder.[1,2] Unipolar depression, also called major depressive disorder, is the most common mental disorder worldwide and a leading cause of disability.[3] Herein, unipolar depression is simply referred to as depression. It is characterised by depressed mood, a loss of interest, or loss of pleasure in daily activities for more than two weeks. Symptoms may also include irritability, changes in weight, sleep, activity, fatigue or loss of energy, loss of concentration, feelings of guilt or worthlessness or suicidality. The depressive episodes are not caused by psychosis, substance abuse or general medical conditions, and they are not explained by specified and unspecified schizophrenia spectrum and psychotic disorders. People with depression do not have a history of mania, or mixed or hypomanic episodes, as people with bipolar disorder do.[4,5] Clinical presentation of depression is heterogeneous. Depression may present as an isolated episode or people may suffer from recurrent episodes,[6,7] but for most people it is a life-long disorder.[1]

# Epidemiology

Depression is the most commonly reported mental disorder worldwide and the World Health Organization (WHO) reports that 151.1 million people are affected. Prevalence is unrelated to age, ethnicity or income.[3] Depression affects people from varying regions and economic profiles, with low-, middle-, and high-income earners affected.[3,8] The adjusted global point prevalence of depression is 4.7%, and it has a 12-month prevalence of 6.6% and a lifetime prevalence of 16.2%.[3,10] Depression is more common in women than men and working adults.[3,10] It is prevalent in all age groups, especially adults and the elderly. However, many people experience their first episode during childhood and adolescence.[5,6]

Each year approximately 16.1 million (6.7%) adults in the United States of America (USA) experience at least one major depressive episode.[11] In Canada, the prevalence of depression is 4.7%[12] and in Europe it affects approximately 33.4 million people.[13] In Australia, 4.1% of adults have had a depressive episode in the past 12 months[14] and one in 11 (8.9%) reported depression or feelings of depression.[15] In China, more than 54 million people, 4.2% of the population, suffer from depression.[16]

## Burden

Depression accounts for approximately 2.5% of the global disability adjusted life years (DALYs).[17] It is projected to be the second leading cause of DALYs by 2030, surpassing previously top ranked diseases such as perinatal conditions and lower respiratory tract infections.[18]

Data also shows that the burden of depression increased by 37.5% between 1990 and 2010, due to population growth and ageing.[17,19] In the USA, depression accounts for 3.7% of all DALYs[11] and accounts for 16 million suicide DALYs when it is considered as a risk factor for suicide.[17] In Europe, depression is the third highest burden of disease and accounts for 3.8% of all DALYs.[16]

Depression is ranked as one of the top causes of global years lived with disability (YLD).[3,11] It accounts for 8.2% (5.9–10.8%) of global YLD.[17] In the USA, depression accounts for 8.3% of all YLD.[11] Between 1990 and 2010 depression has remained the second highest disease, after low back pain, with the largest number of YLD. In high-income countries, depression accounts for 10 million and is 14.6% of total YLD.[3] The yearly YLD associated with depression for males is 24.3 million and 8.3% of total YLD and for females is 41 million and 13.4% of total YLD.[3] With regards to age, YLD peaks in the twenties and gradually decreases with age.

Globally, in 2010 the largest proportion of YLDs from depressive disorders occurred in individuals of working age (15 to 64 years) with 60.4 million YLDs, followed by the zero to 14 years age group with 7.8 million YLDs, and the 65 and over age group with 6.1 million YLDs.[17] Two multi-country projects — the WHO's Study on Global Ageing and Adult Health (SAGE) and the Collaborative Research on Ageing in Europe (COURAGE) showed that domestic life, work and interpersonal activities were the most affected quality of life elements.[20]

In the USA, over 16.1 million adults had at least one major depressive episode in 2013.[11] An average of five weeks of lost work productivity and the annualised human capital loss to employers associated with depression was estimated to be in excess of $36 billion US.[21] The estimated annual medical and workplace costs exceeded $200 billion US in 2010.[22] In Europe, the economic costs of depression amounts to €136.3 billion Euros, including reduced productivity (€99.3 billion) and healthcare system costs (€37 billion).[13,23] In China, a cost of $7.8 billion US is associated with lost work days, medical expenses and funeral expenses every year.[24]

The WHO World Health Survey showed that depression results in the greatest reduction in health compared to chronic diseases including angina, arthritis, asthma, and diabetes. The comorbid state of depression incrementally worsens health scores compared with depression alone, any of the chronic diseases alone, and with any combination of chronic diseases without depression.[25]

In summary, the disease burden of depression is enormous, including functional impairment and reduced quality of life, as well as social and economic costs. Trends show that this burden continues to rise.

## Risk Factors

Risk factors of depression include family history, biological, and environmental factors. The heritability is estimated at 31% to 42%.[26] The biological children (generation 3) of depressed, compared with non-depressed parents (generation 2), have a two-fold increased risk of depression; biological offspring with two previous generations affected with depression are at the highest risk for depression.[27] Non-genetic factors explain 60–70% of the susceptibility to depression.[28] These factors are childhood, or recent, interpersonal adversities including sexual abuse, other lifetime trauma, low social support, marital problems and divorce.[29,30] Depression is twice as common in women as it is in men,[10] also females are more likely to have reoccurring episodes.[7] Although onset can occur at any stage of life, many factors associated with depression are either age specific or age restricted. These include biological events such as puberty, menopause, dementia, chronic diseases, and environmental risk factors including childhood maltreatment, childbirth, and parental divorce.[1,31]

## Pathological Processes

Depression is defined by non-specific behavioural signs and symptoms such as low mood, impaired concentration, insomnia and fatigue, rather than a distinct pathophysiology.[32,33] Currently, there is limited knowledge on the aetiology and pathophysiology of depression.[32,34]

The most commonly studied brain systems in neurobiological research of depression have been the monoaminergic neurotransmitter systems.[34] The monoaminergic systems are extensively distributed throughout the limbic, striatal and prefrontal cortical neuronal circuits.[35-37] In human brain imaging studies and post-mortem studies of patients with depression, these structures and interconnected circuits are implicated in the pathophysiology of depression.[5,33,38,39] These regions regulate learning and contextual memory processes, executive function, emotion and reward, and have been implicated in depression and antidepressant actions.[33] Due to the heterogeneity of the disease, different regions of the brain might be involved in different individuals and different pathophysiologies occur at different stages of the disease.[33]

Brain region involvement in depression stems from some of the key symptoms of the disorder itself, which include dysregulation of circadian rhythms, altered cognitive processing, both appetitive and psychomotor episodes, and high levels of episode-related impairment and functioning.[5] Frontal regions of the cortex and hippocampus might mediate cognitive aspects of depression, such as memory impairment and feelings of worthlessness, hopelessness, guilt, doom, and suicidality.[33] The striatum (particularly the ventral striatum or nucleus accumbens), amygdala, and related brain areas are important in mediating aversive and rewarding responses to emotional stimuli. As a result these regions could mediate the anhedonia, anxiety and reduced motivation that predominates in many patients with depression.[33] The involvement of the hypothalamus has also been suggested as it regulates metabolic and autonomic systems. Abnormalities presented in depressive symptoms, including too much or too little sleep, appetite or energy, as well as a loss of interest in sex and other pleasurable activities, suggests the involvement of the hypothalamus.[33]

Assessments of cerebrospinal fluid chemistry, neuroendocrine responses to pharmacological challenge, and neuroreceptor and transporter binding have demonstrated a number of abnormalities of neurotransmitter and neuropeptide systems in depression. These include the serotonergic, noradrenergic, dopaminergic, cholinergic, glutamatergic, and gamma-aminobutyric acid (GABA)-ergic systems, corticotropin-releasing hormone (CRH) and the hypothalamic-pituitary-adrenal axis.[34]

Connectivity of serotonergic, noradrenergic and dopaminergic neurons occur through neural circuits.[40] A relationship exists between the three main monoamine neurotransmitters in the brain and the symptoms of depression.[41] Norepinephrine is thought to relate to alertness, attention, interest, energy levels, as well as anxiety. Serotonin is related to anxiety, and obsessive and compulsive behaviour while dopamine is related to attention, motivation, pleasure, reward and interest in life.[41] Through different mechanisms, the use of antidepressants results in an increase in concentration of the monoamine neurotransmitters norepinephrine, serotonin and dopamine at the synapse, enhancement of neurotransmission and improvement of the symptoms for depression.

Hormones also play a role in depression. CRH from the hypothalamus is released during times of psychological stress by cortical brain regions.[28,29] It induces the secretion of pituitary corticotropin to stimulate release of cortisol into the plasma by the adrenal gland.[28,29] The presence of CRH produces several physiological and behavioural changes seen in depression including altered appetite, disrupted sleep, decreased libido, and psychomotor alterations.[42] Hypersecretion of CRH has been shown in patient with depression and suggests that CRH may participate in the initiation or perpetuation of the depression cycle.[43]

## Diagnosis

Diagnosis of depression is based on a number of symptomatic criteria including the American Psychiatric Association's Diagnostic and Statistical Manual of Mental Disorders, Fifth Edition (DSM-V)[1] and the World Health Organisation's International Classification of Diseases-10th Revision (ICD-10).[44] Laboratory tests do not provide results of sufficient sensitivity and specificity to be used as a diagnostic tool for depression. A diagnosis based on a single episode can be considered a major depressive episode, but a symptom must be newly present or must be clearly worse compared with the person's pre-episode status.

The following diagnostic criterion for unipolar depression is adapted from the Diagnostic and Statistical Manual of Mental Disorders (DSM)-V:[1]

A. At least five or more of the following symptoms must be present, with depressed mood or decreased interest or pleasure as one of the five, persisting over a two-week period:

   1. Depressed mood most of the day, occurring most days (subjective or observed);
   2. Markedly diminished interest or pleasure most of the day, nearly every day;
   3. Significant weight or appetite change, nearly every day;
   4. Insomnia or hypersomnia, nearly every day;
   5. Psychomotor agitation or retardation (observable by others), nearly every day;
   6. Fatigue or loss of energy, nearly every day;
   7. Feelings of worthlessness or inappropriate guilt, nearly every day;
   8. Diminished ability to concentrate or make decisions, nearly every day;
   9. Recurring thoughts of death or suicide plans.

B. The symptoms cause clinically significant distress or impairment in social, occupational, or other important areas of functioning;
C. The symptoms are not attributed to the physiological effects of a substance (alcohol, medication or street drug) or to another medical condition;
D. The occurrence of the major depressive episode is not due to other psychiatric disorders such as mania, hypomania, bipolar disorder, or schizophrenia;
E. There has never been a manic episode or a hypomanic episode.

Criteria A–C represents a major depressive episode.

Remission is a period of two or more months with no symptoms, or only one or two symptoms to no more than a mild degree (DSM-V).[1] Periods of remission can be partial or full. Following a major depressive episode, if the symptoms of the episode are present but the full criteria of diagnosis are not met, or there is a period lasting less than two months without any significant symptoms of an episode, the patient is in partial remission.[1] If no significant signs or symptoms are detected for two or more months following an episode, the patient is in full remission.[1] Recurrence is defined as the return of depressive symptoms during the maintenance phase, there must be an interval of at least two consecutive months between separate episodes to be considered a new, distinct episode.[1,45]

Depression may also be classified as mild, moderate or severe based on symptoms and functional impairment. For example, mild depression includes distressing symptoms which are manageable, and the symptoms result in minor impairment in social or occupational functioning. Moderate depression presents with symptoms and functional impairment between those of "mild" and "severe". Moderate symptoms may include withdrawal from family, school and work relationships and decreased socialisation. People may also minimise, or deny, any issues, or project onto others or blame others. They may also have vague or occasional suicidal thoughts. Finally, severe depression includes severe functional impairment and withdrawal from social and work activities, psychotic symptoms, recent suicide attempt, or specific suicide plan or clear intent. The number of symptoms is in excess of that required to make the diagnosis, the intensity of the symptoms is seriously distressing and unmanageable, and the symptoms markedly interfere with social and occupational functioning.[1]

When diagnosing depression, special care should be taken to avoid misdiagnosis with other conditions. Persistent depressive disorder is diagnosed when adults with depression present with depressed mood that occurs for most of the day for two years.[1] During the two years, any symptom-free intervals last no longer than two months.[1] Whereas depression can have remission and symptom-free intervals for two months or more. Major depressive episodes occur when life events that represent significant loss, for example bereavement, financial ruin, loses from a natural disaster, a serious medical illness or disability, trigger responses including intense sadness, rumination about the loss, insomnia, poor appetite, and weight loss noted in the diagnostic criteria.[1] The episode resembles a major depressive episode but subsides with time, does not reoccur and may not be diagnosable as depression. Socio-economic factors that cause a major depressive episode can trigger depression. However, some patients with depressive symptoms cannot identify the specific cause(s) for their condition.

# Management

Due to the uniqueness of depression, psychiatric management must be provided during all phases of treatment as patients may self-harm. Before treatment, assessment of suicide risk is essential and can be assessed considering the following factors (adapted from the American Psychiatric Association, Practice Guideline for the Treatment of Patients with Major Depressive Disorder, 2010)[46]:

- Presence of suicidal or homicidal ideation, intent, or plans;
- History and seriousness of previous attempts;
- Access to means for suicide and the lethality of those means;
- Presence of severe anxiety, panic attacks, agitation, and/or impulsivity;
- Presence of psychotic symptoms, such as command hallucinations;
- Poor reality testing;
- Presence of alcohol or other substance use;
- Family history of, or recent exposure to suicide;
- Absence of protective factors.

Please note that this does not predict attempted, or complete, suicide. Close monitoring is required if the patient shows signs of suicide, homicide intention or planning; psychiatric service and/or hospitalisation should be considered if the risk is significant.[46,47] The severity and duration of the depressive symptoms must also be routinely determined.[47] The clinical management of depression focuses on pharmacotherapy and psychotherapy/cognitive behavioural therapy.[48,49] Physical treatments and complementary and alternative treatments can be used,[47] and lifestyle management should also be considered.[50]

## Treatment Phases

The treatment of depression comprises of three phases: acute (6 to 12 weeks), continuation (4 to 9 months), and maintenance (≥1 year).[51,52] After psychological assessment of patients, treatments may be discontinued with ongoing monitoring of symptoms (Table 1.1).

**Table 1.1.    Treatment Phases of Depression**

| Phase | Pre-treatment Assessment | Treatment Goal |
|---|---|---|
| Acute (6–12 weeks) | Suicide risk. | • Induce remission;<br>• Achieve full return of patient's level of functioning prior to the depressive episode. |
| Continuation (4–9 months) | Monitor for signs of relapse. | • Reduce the high risk of relapse;<br>• Continue treatment. |
| Maintenance (≥1 year) | Monitor for signs of recurrence. | • Determine if the patient needs maintenance treatment. |
| Discontinuation | For stable patients, consider discontinuation of treatment. | |
| Monitoring | Systematic assessment. | • Monitor for potential relapse;<br>• Schedule follow-up visit. |

## Acute Phase Treatment

The aim of acute phase treatment is to induce remission of the major depressive episode and achieve full return to the patient's level of functioning prior to the episode.[46] Treatment selection is based on severity of the depressive symptoms and may vary depending on patients' preferences. Factors affecting treatment selection include specific psychosocial stressors, medical conditions, healthcare expenses, and previous experience.

For individuals diagnosed with mild depression, first-line treatments include psycho-education, self-management, and psychological treatments.[46] In some cases, pharmacological treatments can be considered when there is patient preference, previous response to antidepressants, or lack of response to non-pharmacological interventions.[53] First-line treatment recommendations for moderate depression include second-generation antidepressant monotherapy, psychotherapy, and a combination of both.[53] Pharmacotherapy is preferred when there is prior positive response to an antidepressant, significant sleep or appetite disturbance or agitation, patients preference, and anticipation of a need for maintenance therapy.[46] Severe depression may require the combination of an antidepressant and antipsychotic, electroconvulsive therapy, or the combination of an antidepressant and psychotherapy.[53]

## Continuation Phase Treatment

After the patient has received treatment in the acute phase and has resumed their level of functioning to that experienced prior to the episode, the next phase aims to reduce the high-risk of relapse and continues treatment. Approximately 85% of people who recover from a major depressive episode will experience a second episode within 15 years.[7] Relapse is defined as the return of depressive symptoms during the acute, or continuation, phases and is therefore considered part of the same depressive episode.[45] Antidepressants can be used for 4 to 9 months at the same dosage used to achieve remission in the acute phase.[46] Signs of relapse can be monitored by systematic assessment of depressive symptoms, functional status and quality of life; patients and families can also help identify signs of relapse.[46]

## Maintenance Phase Treatment

This phase will determine if the patient requires maintenance treatment. Recurrence is defined as the return of depressive symptoms during the maintenance phase, there must be an interval of at least two consecutive months between separate episodes to be considered a new, distinct episode.[1,45] The risk of recurrence is 50% after the recovery from the first episode.[46,54] Maintenance therapy should be considered for patients who have had three or more prior episodes, or chronic and recurring illness.[46] The same effective treatment in the acute and continuation phase should be used during the maintenance phase, and patients should be monitored systematically and at regular intervals.[46]

## Discontinuation of Treatment and Monitoring

Currently there are no guidelines or systematic studies on when and how to discontinue treatment for depression. Clinically, certain factors may be considered when discontinuing treatment which include the likelihood of recurrence based on previous episodes, characteristics of previous episodes such as frequency and severity, any residual depressive symptoms after remission, other comorbidities, as well as patient choice.[46] It is often recommended that stopping pharmacotherapy should be gradual and recurring symptoms should be monitored to avoid symptoms such as nausea, headache, chills, and body aches.[46] As depression is a lifelong condition, the patient should be monitored and a plan for returning to treatment when required.

## Pharmacological Treatments

The use of antidepressants is determined by the duration and severity of depression. It is the first-line of treatment for moderate and severe major depressive patients but not recommended for mild episodes of depression, nor in children or adolescents.[47] First-generation antidepressants include tricyclic antidepressants (TCAs) and monoamine oxidase inhibitors (MAOIs); second-generation antidepressants include selective serotonin reuptake inhibitors (SSRIs), serotonin norepinephrine reuptake inhibitors (SNRIs) and bupropion (Table 1.2).[46] Nowadays, first-generation antidepressants are rarely used, for most patients second-generation antidepressants are used and are optimal in terms of safety and efficacy.[46]

There are different patterns of side effects between groups of antidepressants: TCAs and noradrenaline reuptake inhibitors include antimuscarinic side effects, dizziness and sweating; SSRIs/SNRIs have gastrointestinal, stimulatory and sexual side effects; mirtazapine can cause sedation and weight gain.[47] TCAs and MAOIs have greater toxicity and potential to cause death via overdose than SSRIs and most

**Table 1.2. Pharmacological Treatments for Depression**

| Drug Class (Mechanism of Action) | Drugs | Usual Dose (mg/day) |
|---|---|---|
| Selective serotonin reuptake inhibitors (selectively inhibits the reuptake of serotonin) | Citalopram | 20–60 |
| | Escitalopram | 10–20 |
| | Fluoxetine | 20–60 |
| | Paroxetine | 20–60 |
| | Paroxetine, extended release | 25–75 |
| | Sertraline | 50–200 |
| | Fluoxetine | 20–60 |
| Tricyclic antidepressants (non-selectively inhibits the reuptake of monoamines including serotonin, dopamine, and norepinephrine) | Amitriptyline 25–50, 100–300 | 100–300 |
| | Doxepin | 100–300 |
| | Imipramine | 100–300 |
| | Desipramine | 100–300 |
| | Nortriptyline | 50–200 |
| | Trimipramine | 75–300 |
| | Protriptyline | 20–60 |
| | Maprotiline | 100–225 |
| Norepinephrine-dopamine reuptake inhibitor (inhibits the reuptake of norepinephrine and dopamine) | Bupropion, immediate release | 300–450 |
| | Bupropion, sustained release | 300–400 |
| | Bupropion, extended release | 300–450 |
| Serotonin modulator (primarily antagonises 5-HT$_2$ receptors) | Nefazodone | 150–300 |
| | Trazodone | 150–600 |
| Serotonin-norepinephrine reuptake inhibitors (inhibits the reuptake of serotonin and norepinephrine) | Venlafaxine, immediate release | 75–375 |
| | Venlafaxine, extended release | 75–375 |
| | Desvenlafaxine | 50 |
| | Duloxetine | 60–120 |
| Noradrenergic and specific serotonergic modulators (primarily antagonises adrenergic α-2 receptors and 5-HT$_{2C}$ receptors) | Mirtazapine | 15–45 |
| Monoamine oxidase inhibitors (non-selectively inhibits enzymes [MAO-A and MAO-B] involved | Phenelzine | 45–90 |
| | Tranylcypromine | 30–60 |

*(Continued)*

**Table 1.2.** (*Continued*)

| Drug Class (Mechanism of Action) | Drugs | Usual Dose (mg/day) |
|---|---|---|
| in the breakdown of monoamines, including serotonin, dopamine, and norepinephrine MAO-B selective inhibitor) | Isocarboxazid | 30–60 |
| | Selegiline transdermal | 6–12 |
| | Moclobemide | 300–600 |
| Serotonin reuptake inhibitor and 5-HT$_{1A}$-receptor partial agonist (potently, and selectively, inhibits serotonin reuptake and acts as a partial agonist at the 5-HT$_{1A}$ receptor) | Vilazodone | 20–40 |

Antidepressant drug classes and dosing information adapted from Kupfer *et al.*, 2012, and APA, 2010.[10,44]

Abbreviations: 5-HT, serotonin; MAO, Monoamine oxidase.

other new antidepressants, such as the use of MAOIs is restricted to patients who do not respond to other treatments.[46,47]

## Non-pharmacological Treatments

There are several types of non-pharmacological treatments for depression, including psychological and behavioral treatments, physical treatments, and complementary treatments. For depression that is mild to moderate in severity, cognitive behavioral therapy, activity scheduling, and interpersonal psychotherapy are alternatives to antidepressants in acute treatment.[47] Cognitive behavioural therapy is recommended if psychological treatment is used as monotherapy for recurrent depression. Cognitive behavioural therapy includes face-to-face (individual or group) or online behavioural, cognitive, and educational components to help people develop healthy habits and skills to improve their depression and associated symptoms, such as sleep. For severe major depression, psychological or behavioural treatment conducted by an experienced therapist is routinely considered as an add-on therapy to antidepressant treatment.[47]

Electroconvulsive therapy is considered as a first-line treatment for severe depression in the emergency situation (e.g. not eating or drinking, depressive stupor, extreme distress) and when depression is accompanied by melancholia, psychotic features, and/or suicidality.[47,55] Current recommendation is to consider unilateral electroconvulsive therapy initially to minimise adverse cognitive effects.[55] For the acute treatment of seasonal (autumn/winter) depression, light therapy is the first-line treatment with effective prophylaxis against relapse, along with antidepressants.[46] St. John's Wort and omega-3 fatty acids are complementary treatments that have been used for depression.[47,55]

## Prevention

Prevention of depression has been recognised since the 1990s.[56] Research indicates that there is a 21% decrease in depression in people undertaking prevention strategies, compared to people using psychological interventions.[57] Therefore, effective prevention of the disease can delay or prevent the onset of depression in new patients, in turn, reducing disease burden and economic costs.[57]

Being a disease of high recurrence and relapse, identifying risk factors can also be effective in preventing recurrence and relapse. In the primary care and specialised mental healthcare settings, subclinical residual symptoms and the number of previous episodes are the most important predictors for recurrence of depression, whereas demographic factors are not related to recurrence of depression.[58] The most important risk factors for relapse are presence of residual symptoms, number of previous episodes, severity, duration, and degree of treatment resistance of the most recent episode.[47]

## Prognosis

Depression is a lifetime and recurrent disease.[20] It may affect people at any age, and onset of disease may be associated with puberty or major life events. The course of depression is variable, some individuals rarely experience remission while others experience many years with few or no symptoms between discrete episodes.[1] Recovery typically begins within three months of onset for two out of every five individuals, and within one year for four out of every five individuals.[1] After recovery from the first major depressive episode, the risk of recurrence is at least 50%.[46,54] Strategies to prevent recurrence of a depressive episode can be highly effective.[58]

# References

1. American Psychiatric Association. (2013) Diagnostic and Statistical Manual of Mental Disorders, 5th ed. American Psychiatric Association, Arlington, VA.
2. Shahrokh NC, Hales RE, Phillips KA, and Yudofsky SC. (2011) The Language of Mental Health: A Glossary of Psychiatric Terms. American Psychiatric Publishing, Inc, Washington, DC.
3. World Health Organization. (2004) The Global Burden of Disease: 2004 update Part 3: Disease Incidence, Prevalence and Disability.
4. Belmaker RH and Agam G. (2008) Major depressive disorder. *N Engl J Med* **358**(1): 55–68.
5. Fava M and Kendler KS. (2000) Major depressive disorder. *Neuron* **28**(2): 335–341.
6. Kessler RC, Akiskal HS, Ames M, *et al.* (2009) The global burden of mental disorders: An update from the WHO World Mental Health (WMH) Surveys. *Epidemiol Psichiatr Soc* **18**(1): 23–33.
7. Mueller TI, Leon AC, Keller MB, *et al.* (1999) Recurrence after recovery from major depressive disorder during 15 years of observational follow-up. *Am J Psychiatry* **156**(7): 1000–1006.
8. Alonso J, Petukhova M, Vilagut G, *et al.* (2011) Days out of role due to common physical and mental conditions: results from the WHO World Mental Health surveys. *Mol Psychiatry* **16**(12): 1234–1246.
9. Ferrari AJ, Somerville AJ, Baxter AJ, *et al.* (2013) Global variation in the prevalence and incidence of major depressive disorder: a systematic review of the epidemiological literature. *Psychol Med* **43**(3): 471–481.
10. Kupfer DJ, Frank E, and Phillips ML. (2012) Major depressive disorder: new clinical, neurobiological, and treatment perspectives. *Lancet* **379**(9820): 1045–1055.
11. National Institute of Health. Center for Behavioral Health Statistics and Quality. (2016) 2015 National Survey on Drug Use and Health: Major Depression Among Adults. Substance Abuse and Mental Health

Services Administration, Rockville, MD. Available from: https://www.nimh.nih.gov/health/statistics/prevalence/major-depression-among-adults.shtml.

12. Patten SB, Williams JV, Lavorato DH, *et al.* (2015) Descriptive epidemiology of major depressive disorder in Canada in 2012. *Can J Psychiatry* **60**(1): 23–30.

13. Smit F, Shields L, and Petrea I. (2016) Preventing Depression in the WHO European Region. WHO Regional Office for Europe.

14. Australian Bureau of Statistics. (2008) National Survey of Mental Health and Wellbeing: Summary of Results, 2007. Australia, ABS cat. no. 4326.0. Canberra.

15. Australian Bureau of Statistics. (2015) National Health Survey: First Results, 2014–15. Australia, ABS cat. no. 4364.0.55.001. Canberra.

16. World Health Organisation. (2014) Global Health Estimates 2014 Summary Tables: DALY by cause, age and sex, by WHO Region, 2000–2012. Available from: http://www.euro.who.int/en/health-topics/noncommunicable-diseases/mental-health/data-and-statistics.

17. Ferrari AJ, Charlson FJ, Norman RE, *et al.* (2013) Burden of depressive disorders by country, sex, age, and year: findings from the global burden of disease study 2010. *PLoS Med* **10**(11): e1001547.

18. Mathers CD and Loncar D. (2006) Projections of global mortality and burden of disease from 2002 to 2030. *PLoS Med* **3**(11): e442.

19. Murray CJ and Lopez AD. (1996) Evidence-based health policy — lessons from the Global Burden of Disease Study. *Science* **274**(5288): 740–743.

20. Kamenov K, Caballero FF, Miret M, *et al.* (2016) Which Are the Most Burdensome Functioning Areas in Depression? A Cross-National Study. *Front Psychol* **7**: 1342.

21. Kessler RC, Akiskal HS, Ames M, *et al.* (2006) Prevalence and effects of mood disorders on work performance in a nationally representative sample of U.S. workers. *Am J Psychiatry* **163**(9): 1561–1568.

22. Greenberg PE, Fournier AA, Sisitsky T, *et al.* (2015) The economic burden of adults with major depressive disorder in the United States (2005 and 2010). *J Clin Psychiatry* **76**(2): 155–162.

23. Andlin-Sobocki P, Jonsson B, Wittchen HU, *et al.* (2005) Cost of disorders of the brain in Europe. *Eur J Neurol* **12**(Suppl 1): 1–27.

24. World Health Organisation. (2017) WHO China Office Fact Sheet: Depression. Available from: http://www.wpro.who.int/china/topics/mental_health/20170331_factsheet_depression_eng.pdf.

25. Moussavi S, Chatterji S, Verdes E, *et al.* (2007) Depression, chronic diseases, and decrements in health: results from the World Health Surveys. *Lancet* **370**(9590): 851–858.

26. Sullivan PF, Neale MC, and Kendler KS. (2000) Genetic epidemiology of major depression: review and meta-analysis. *Am J Psychiatry* **157**(10): 1552–1562.

27. Weissman MM, Berry OO, Warner V, *et al.* (2016) A 30-Year Study of 3 Generations at High Risk and Low Risk For Depression. *JAMA Psychiatry* **73**(9): 970–977.

28. Hasler G. (2010) Pathophysiology of depression: do we have any solid evidence of interest to clinicians? *World Psychiatry* **9**(3): 155–161.

29. Kendler KS, Sheth K, Gardner CO, *et al.* (2002) Childhood parental loss and risk for first-onset of major depression and alcohol dependence: the time-decay of risk and sex differences. *Psychol Med* **32**(7): 1187–1194.

30. Kendler KS, Gardner CO, and Prescott CA. (2006) Toward a comprehensive developmental model for major depression in men. *Am J Psychiatry* **163**(1): 115–124.

31. Power RA, Tansey KE, Buttenschon HN, *et al.* (2017) Genome-wide Association for Major Depression Through Age at Onset Stratification: Major Depressive Disorder Working Group of the Psychiatric Genomics Consortium. *Biol Psychiatry* **81**(4): 325–335.

32. Drevets WC. (2001) Neuroimaging and neuropathological studies of depression: implications for the cognitive-emotional features of mood disorders. *Curr Opin Neurobiol* **11**(2): 240–249.

33. Berton O, McClung CA, Dileone RJ, *et al.* (2006) Essential role of BDNF in the mesolimbic dopamine pathway in social defeat stress. *Science* **311**(5762): 864–868.

34. Manji HK, Drevets WC, and Charney DS. (2001) The cellular neurobiology of depression. *Nat Med* **7**(5): 541–547.

35. Drevets WC. (2000) Functional anatomical abnormalities in limbic and prefrontal cortical structures in major depression. *Prog Brain Res* **126**: 413–431.

36. Graybiel AM. (1990) Neurotransmitters and neuromodulators in the basal ganglia. *Trends Neurosci* **13**(7): 244–254.

37. Drevets WC. (1999) Prefrontal cortical-amygdalar metabolism in major depression. *Ann N Y Acad Sci* **877**: 614–637.

38. Price JL and Drevets WC. (2012) Neural circuits underlying the pathophysiology of mood disorders. *Trends Cogn Sci* **16**(1): 61–71.

39. Chiriţă AL, Gheorman V, Bondari D, *et al*. (2015) Current understanding of the neurobiology of major depressive disorder. *Rom J Morphol Embryol* **56**(2 Suppl): 651–658.
40. Hamon M and Blier P. (2013) Monoamine neurocircuitry in depression and strategies for new treatments. *Prog Neuropsychopharmacol Biol Psychiatry* **45**: 54–63.
41. Nutt DJ. (2008) Relationship of neurotransmitters to the symptoms of major depressive disorder. *J Clin Psychiatry* **69** (Suppl E1): 4–7.
42. Nemeroff CB. (1996) The corticotropin-releasing factor (CRF) hypothesis of depression: new findings and new directions. *Mol Psychiatry* **1**(4): 336–342.
43. Tsigos C and Chrousos GP. (2002) Hypothalamic-pituitary-adrenal axis, neuroendocrine factors and stress. *J Psychosom Res* **53**(4): 865–871.
44. World Health Organisation. (1993) International Classification of Diseases (ICD-10) World Health Organisation, Geneva, Switzerland.
45. Qaseem A, Barry MJ, and Kansagara D. (2016) Nonpharmacologic Versus Pharmacologic Treatment of Adult Patients With Major Depressive Disorder: A Clinical Practice Guideline From the American College of Physicians. *Ann Intern Med* **164**(5): 350–359.
46. American Psychiatric Association. (2010) Practice Guideline for the Treatment of Patients With Major Depressive Disorder.
47. Anderson IM, Ferrier IN, Baldwin RC, *et al*. (2008) Evidence-based guidelines for treating depressive disorders with antidepressants: a revision of the 2000 British Association for Psychopharmacology guidelines. *J Psychopharmacol* **22**(4): 343–396.
48. Malhi GS, Hitching R, Berk M, *et al*. (2013) Pharmacological management of unipolar depression. *Acta Psychiatr Scand* Suppl (443): 6–23.
49. Lampe L, Coulston CM, and Berk L. (2013) Psychological management of unipolar depression. *Acta Psychiatr Scand* Suppl (443): 24–37.
50. Berk M, Sarris J, Coulson CE, *et al*. (2013) Lifestyle management of unipolar depression. *Acta Psychiatr Scand* Suppl (443): 38–54.
51. Kupfer DJ, Perel JM, Pollock BG, *et al*. (1991) Fluvoxamine versus desipramine: comparative polysomnographic effects. *Biol Psychiatry* **29**(1): 23–40.
52. Gartlehner G, Gaynes BN, Amick HR, *et al*. (2015) Nonpharmacological Versus Pharmacological Treatments for Adult Patients With Major Depressive Disorder, RTI International-University of North Carolina Evidence-based Practice Center Research Triangle Park, NC.

53. Davidson JR. (2010) Major depressive disorder treatment guidelines in America and Europe. *J Clin Psychiatry* **71** (Suppl E1): e04.
54. Kupfer DJ, Frank E, and Wamhoff J. (1996) Mood disorders: Update on prevention of recurrence. In: Mundt C, Goldstein MJ, editors. (1996). Interpersonal factors in the origin and course of affective disorders. London, England: Gaskell/Royal College of Psychiatrists; 1996. pp. 289–302.
55. Ellis P. (2004) Australian and New Zealand clinical practice guidelines for the treatment of depression. *Aust N Z J Psychiatry* **38**(6): 389–407.
56. Institute of Medicine Committee on Prevention of Mental Disorders. (1994) Reducing Risks for Mental Disorders: Frontiers for Preventive Intervention Research. PJ Mrazek and RJ Haggerty, Washington (DC), National Academies Press (US).
57. van Zoonen K, Buntrock C, Ebert DD, *et al.* (2014) Preventing the onset of major depressive disorder: a meta-analytic review of psychological interventions. *Int J Epidemiol* **43**(2): 318–329.
58. Hardeveld F, Spijker J, De Graaf R, *et al.* (2013) Recurrence of major depressive disorder across different treatment settings: results from the NESDA study. *J Affect Disord* **147**(1–3): 225–231.

# 2

# Unipolar Depression in Chinese Medicine

## OVERVIEW

In Chinese medicine, unipolar depression is commonly known as *yu bing* 郁病, and also relates to other Chinese medicine diseases and syndromes, such as *bei die* 卑慄, *bai he bing* 百合病, *zang zao* 脏躁, *mei he qi* 梅核气, *shi zhi* 失志, and *ben tun qi* 奔豚气. Chinese medicine theory states that depression is located in the Liver and related to the Heart, Spleen, and Kidney. This chapter introduces the main etiology, pathogenesis and syndromes of depression in Chinese Medicine. Treatments are described based on Chinese medicine textbooks, clinical practice and principles and guidelines, including Chinese herbal medicine, acupuncture, and diet therapy.

## Introduction

Unipolar depression, also referred to as major depressive disorder, is a modern disease name that cannot be identified as a specific Chinese medicine (CM) disease. This is due to different theoretical systems between conventional medicine and CM, and different ways of understanding diseases. Although CM does not specify unipolar depression, there has been a considerable amount of disease description of depression since the Spring and Autumn periods of China (770–476 BC). For example, the book *Chu Ci* 楚辞 states that people may *"feel depressed and frustrated"*. The word depression is also found in the classical medical book, the *Huang Di Nei Jing* 黄帝内经 (written before AD 618), including related terms such as sad, unhappy, and worry. The *Huang Di Nei Jing* 黄帝内经 also described the negative effects of these emotions on one's well-being. Modern CM practitioners and scholars consider depression being mainly related to *yu bing* 郁病, but that can also be found in other CM diseases and symptoms, such as *bei die* 卑慄, *bai he bing* 百合病, *zang zao* 脏躁, *mei he qi* 梅核气, *shi zhi* 失志, and *ben tun qi* 奔豚气.[1-7]

## Aetiology and Pathogenesis

Based on traditional CM theory, depression is caused by the seven emotions and emotional frustration, which results in an imbalance of internal organs, *yin* and *yang*, and *qi* and Blood, leading to malnourishment of the *shen* 神 (mind). Depression is located in the Liver and related to the Heart, Spleen, and Kidney. When the seven emotions are in excess, it may cause diseases. For example, excessive anger injures the Liver which leads to Liver *qi* stagnation, while excessive thinking injures the Spleen and causes stagnation of Spleen *qi*, resulting in stagnant *qi* transforming into Phlegm. If Liver *qi* is stagnant, it may overact and impair the Spleen, resulting in a disharmony of the Liver and Spleen. Stagnant Liver *qi* can transform into Fire leading to hyperactive Heart Fire. In addition, Liver Fire can impair the *yin*, causing malnourishment of the Heart and draining excessively from the Kidney, causing *yin* deficient Fire or Heart and Kidney *yin* deficiency. Stagnant *qi* may result in phlegm-dampness, and stagnant Liver *qi* may transform into fire. When Liver fire is combined with dampness, turning into damp-heat, it may accumulate in the Liver and Gallbladder. Long-term stagnation of *qi* will affect the Blood, leading to Blood stasis. Also, when the Spleen is deficient, there is insufficient generation of *qi* and Blood. When *qi* and Blood are deficient, the Heart and mind are not nourished, resulting in melancholy disturbing the mind, or deficiency of both the Heart and Spleen. The early stages of pathogenesis of depression is excess with stagnation of *qi*, Blood, dampness, phlegm, fire, and food. As for long-term, there is deficiency, or a complex syndrome of deficiency and excess.[1,3]

# Syndrome Differentiation and Treatments

To guide clinical practice, several references can be used that describe CM syndrome differentiation for depression. The Internal Medicine Branch of the China Association of Chinese Medicine (中华中医药学会内科分会) developed Standards for the Diagnosis, Syndrome Differentiation and Evaluation of the Clinical Effect for Depression.[1] This guideline bases treatment on syndrome differentiation. The China Academy of Chinese Medical Sciences (中国中医科学院) developed a CM evidence-based clinical practice guideline according to findings of clinical trials for depression, as well as practitioners' experience. Although this guideline is not the standard for CM treatment for depression, it includes important suggestions and evaluation of efficacy of CM based on current research evidence.[2] On the basis of existing standards and expert consensus, there is the Guideline for the Prevention and Treatment of Depression in China (中国抑郁障碍防治指南).[8] These guidelines are the main references for practitioners in China, in terms of syndrome differentiation and treatments.

The basic treatment principles of CM for depression are to regulate *qi* and soothe *qi* movement, treating with both elimination and reinforcement. When treating excess, it is important to regulate *qi* and activate Blood, purge fire, resolve phlegm, dispel dampness, and promote digestion according to the underlying cause of stagnation, such as *qi*, Blood, dampness, phlegm, fire or food. In addition, attention should be paid to regulating *qi* rather than consuming *qi*, activating Blood rather than impairing Blood, clearing fire rather than injuring the Spleen and Stomach, and expelling phlegm rather than damaging healthy *qi*. As for deficiency syndrome, tonification should be based on the affected internal *zang fu* organs, *qi*, Blood, *yin*, and *yang*, using various treatment methods, including nourishing the Heart and calming the mind, tonifying the Spleen and Stomach, and enriching and nourishing the Liver and Kidney. In terms of combined deficiency-excess syndrome, both deficiency and excess should be taken into consideration and treated according to the severity of the deficiency and excess.[1,3]

## Treatment Based on Syndrome Differentiation

The following syndromes and Chinese herbal medicine (CHM) treatments for depression are based on the Guideline for Diagnosis and Treatment of Common Internal Diseases in Chinese Medicine-Symptoms of Modern Medicine,[1] the Evidence-based Clinical Practice Guideline of Chinese Medicine,[2] and the Chinese Internal Medicine Textbook.[3] Summary of syndromes and CHM treatments is presented in Table 2.1.

**Table 2.1.  Summary of Chinese Herbal Medicines for Depression**

| Syndrome Differentiation | Treatment Principle | Formula(e) |
| --- | --- | --- |
| Liver *qi* stagnation | Soothe the Liver, regulate *qi,* and soothe the Middle *Jiao* (Spleen and Stomach). | Modified *Chai hu shu gan san* 柴胡疏肝散加减, or *Xiao yao wan* 逍遥丸, or *Yue ju wan* 越鞠丸 |
| Liver *qi* stagnation and phlegm stagnation | Move *qi*, resolve phlegm, and clear heat. | Modified *Ban xia hou po tang* 半夏厚朴汤加减, or if combined with phlegm-heat, use modified *Wen dan tang* 温胆汤加减 |
| Liver *qi* stagnation and Spleen *qi* deficiency | Soothe the Liver and tonify the Spleen, resolve phlegm and dissipate stagnation. | Modified *Xiao yao san* combined with *Ban xia hou po tang* 逍遥散合半夏厚朴汤加减 |
| *Qi* stagnation transforming into fire | Soothe the Liver and regulate *qi*, clear the Liver and purge fire. | Modified *Dan zhi xiao yao san* 丹栀逍遥散加减 |
| *Qi* stagnation with Blood stasis | Regulate *qi*, activate Blood, and resolve stasis. | Modified *Tong qiao huo xue tang* combined with *Si ni san* 通窍活血汤合四逆散加减, or modified *Xue fu zhu yu tang* 血府逐瘀汤加减 |
| Liver-Gallbladder damp-heat | Clear the Liver and drain the Gallbladder. | Modified *Long dan xie gan tang* 龙胆泻肝汤加减 |
| *Yin* deficiency with fire | Clear heat and soothe the Liver, enrich the Kidney and nourish *yin*. | Modified *Zi shui qin gan yin* 滋水清肝饮加减 |
| Deficiency of the Heart and Spleen | Tonify the Spleen and nourish the Heart, tonify *qi* and Blood. | Modified *Gui pi tang* 归脾汤加减 |

**Table 2.1.** (*Continued*)

| Syndrome Differentiation | Treatment Principle | Formula(e) |
|---|---|---|
| Heart and Kidney *yin* deficiency | Tonify the Heart and Kidney *yin*. | Modified *Tian wang bu xin dan* combined with *Liu wei di huang wan* 天王补心丹合六味地黄丸加减 |
| Melancholy disturbing the mind | Nourish the Heart to calm the mind, moisten and release tension with sweet herbs. | Modified *Gan mai da zao tang* 甘麦大枣汤加减 |

# Liver *Qi* Stagnation

Clinical manifestations: Depressed mood, emotional instability, irritability, chest tightness, hypochondriac distension and pain, abdominal distension, belching, loss of appetite, irregular bowel motions, thin and greasy tongue coating, and string-like pulse.

Treatment principle: Soothe the Liver and regulate *qi*.

Formula: Modified *Chai hu shu gan san* 柴胡疏肝散加减;[1,3] *Xiao yao wan* 逍遥丸, or *Yue ju wan* 越鞠丸.[2]

Herbs: *Chai hu* 柴胡, *xiang fu* 香附, *zhi ke* 枳壳, *chen pi* 陈皮, *yu jin* 郁金, *qing pi* 青皮, *zi su geng* 紫苏梗, *he huan pi* 合欢皮, *chuan xiong* 川芎, *shao yao* 芍药, and *gan cao* 甘草.

Main actions of herbs: *Chai hu, xiang fu,* and *zhi ke* soothe the Liver, regulate *qi* and soothe the middle *jiao* (Spleen and Stomach). *Yu jin, qing pi, zi su geng,* and *he huan pi* regulate *qi*. *Chuan xiong* regulates *qi* and activates Blood. *Shao yao* and *gan cao* soothe the Liver and release tension. *Gan cao* harmonises all herbs.

# Liver *Qi* Stagnation and Phlegm Stagnation

Clinical manifestations: Depressed mood, chest tightness, hypochondriac distension, globus hystericus, white greasy tongue coating, and string-like and slippery pulse. Phlegm-heat manifestations include vomiting and nausea, bitter taste in the mouth, yellow and greasy tongue coating, and string-like and slippery pulse.

Treatment principle: Regulate *qi* and resolve phlegm. If heat is present, clear heat.

Formula: Modified *Ban xia hou po tang* 半夏厚朴汤加减,[2,3] or if combined with phlegm-heat, use modified *Wen dan tang* 温胆汤加减.[2]

Herbs: *Ban xia* 半夏, *hou po* 厚朴, *zi su* 紫苏, *fu ling* 茯苓, *sheng jiang* 生姜, *zhu ru* 竹茹, *zhi shi* 枳实, *chen pi* 陈皮, and *gan cao* 甘草.

Main actions of herbs: *Hou po*, *zi su* regulate *qi*, soothe the chest, and soothe the Middle Jiao (Spleen and Stomach). *Ban xia* and *sheng jiang* resolve phlegm, dissipate stagnation, and harmonise the Stomach and direct *qi* downward. The combined use of *ban xia* and *zhu ru*, which are warm and cool, stops vomiting and relieves irritability. C*hen pi* regulates *qi*, moves stagnation, dries dampness and resolves phlegm. *Zhi shi* directs *qi* downward, removes stagnation, relieves phlegm and fullness. The combination of *chen pi* and *zhi shi*, which are warm and cool, regulates *qi* and resolves phlegm. *Fu ling* tonifies the Spleen and drains dampness to cut off the source of phlegm.

## Liver *Qi* Stagnation and Spleen *Qi* Deficiency

Clinical manifestations: Depressed mood, chest tightness, hypochondriac distension, abdominal distension and belching, excessive thinking, feelings of uncertainty, worry, sighing, loss of appetite, weight loss, fatigue (especially after activities), menstrual irregularity, irregular bowel motions, thin and greasy tongue coating, and fine and string-like pulse or string-like and slippery pulse.

Treatment principle: Soothe the Liver, tonify the Spleen, resolve phlegm and dissipate stagnation.

Formula: Modified *Xiao yao san* combined with *Ban xia hou po tang* 逍遥散合半夏厚朴汤加减.[1]

Herbs: *Chai hu* 柴胡, *dang gui* 当归, *shao yao* 芍药, *bai zhu* 白术, *gan cao* 甘草, *ban xia* 半夏, *hou po* 厚朴, *fu ling* 茯苓, *sheng jiang* 生姜, and *zi su* 紫苏.

Main actions of herbs: *Chai hu* soothes the Liver and regulates *qi*. *Dang gui* nourishes and harmonises Blood. *Bai shao* nourishes Blood, replenishes *yin*, soothes the Liver and releases tension. *Bai zhu* and *fu ling* tonify the Spleen and dispel dampness. *Gan cao* tonifies *qi* and the middle, soothes the Liver and releases tension. *Sheng jiang* warms the Stomach and harmonises the middle. *Hou po* and *zi su* regulate *qi* and soothe the middle. *Ban xia*, *fu ling*, and *sheng jiang* resolve phlegm, dissipate stagnation, harmonise the Stomach and direct *qi* downward.

## *Qi* Stagnation Transforming into Fire

Clinical manifestations: Emotional irritability, impatience and easily angered, chest and hypochondriac fullness, dry bitter taste in the mouth or headache, red eyes, and tinnitus; or, epigastric distress, acid regurgitation, constipation, red tongue and yellow tongue coating, string-like and rapid pulse.

Treatment principle: Soothe the Liver, regulate *qi* and purge fire.

Formula: Modified *Dan zhi xiao yao san* 丹栀逍遥散(《内科摘要》)加减.[2,3]

Herbs: *Chai hu* 柴胡, *bo he* 薄荷, *yu jin* 郁金, *xiang fu* 香附, *dang gui* 当归, *shao yao* 芍药, *bai zhu* 白术, *fu ling* 茯苓, *mu dan pi* 牡丹皮, and *zhi zi* 栀子.

Main action of herbs: *Chai hu*, *bo he*, *yu jin*, and *xiang fu* soothe the Liver and regulate *qi*. *Dang gui* and *bai shao* tonify Blood and soothe the Liver. *Bai zhu* and *fu ling* tonify the Spleen and dispel dampness. *Mu dan pi* and *zhi zi* regulate the Liver *qi* and purge heat.

### *Qi* Stagnation with Blood Stasis

Clinical manifestations: Depressed mood, irritability, headache, insomnia, forgetfulness, hypochondriac distension and pain, feelings of heat or cold in certain parts of the body, purple tongue with petechia and ecchymosis (red or purple spots or patches) and string-like or rough pulse.

Treatment principle: Regulate *qi*, activate Blood and resolve stasis.

Formula: Modified *Tong qiao huo xue tang* combined with *Si ni san* 通窍活血汤合四逆散加减;[1] or modified *Xue fu zhu yu tang* 血府逐瘀汤加减.[2]

Herbs: *Tao ren* 桃仁, *hong hua* 红花, *dang gui* 当归, *sheng di huang* 生地黄, *niu xi* 牛膝, *chuan xiong* 川芎, *chi shao* 赤芍, *chai hu* 柴胡, *zhi ke* 枳壳, *jie geng* 桔梗, and *gan cao* 甘草.

Main action of herbs: *Tao ren* breaks up Blood stagnation and moistens dryness. *Hong hua* activates Blood and dispels stasis to relieve pain. *Chi shao*, *chuan xiong*, and *niu xi* activate Blood, unblock the meridians, and dispel stasis to relieve pain. *Sheng di huang* and *dang gui* tonify Blood, replenish *yin*, clear heat and activate Blood. *Chai hu* soothes the Liver and regulates *qi*. *Jie geng* soothes chest and regulates *qi*. *Chai hu*, *jie geng*, and *zhi ke* regulate *qi* and move stagnation to promote the movement of *qi* and Blood. *Gan cao* harmonises all herbs.

## Liver-Gallbladder Damp-heat

Clinical manifestations: Depressed mood, or emotional irritability, insomnia with dream-disturbed sleep, hypochondriac distension, bitter taste in the mouth and loss of appetite, vomiting and nausea, fullness in the epigastrium, irregular bowel motions, reddish-yellow urine, red tongue and yellow greasy tongue coating, and string-like, slippery, and rapid pulse.

Treatment principle: Clear the Liver and drain the Gallbladder, clear damp-heat and nourish the Heart to calm the mind.

Formula: Modified *Long dan xie gan tang* 龙胆泻肝汤加减.[1]

Herbs: *Long dan cao* 龙胆草, *zhi zi* 栀子, *huang qin* 黄芩, *mu tong* 木通, *ze xie* 泽泻, *che qian zi* 车前子, *chai hu* 柴胡, *gan cao* 甘草, *dang gui* 当归, *sheng di huang* 生地黄.

Main action of herbs: *Long dan cao* clears the Liver, drains the Gallbladder, and clears damp-heat in the Liver meridian. *Huang qin* and *zhi zi* dry dampness and clear heat. *Ze xie, mu tong,* and *che qian zi* drain dampness, purge heat, and conduct fire back to its origin. *Dang gui* and *sheng di huang* nourish Blood and enrich *yin,* which leads to the removal of unhealthy *qi* without impairing *yin* and Blood. *Chai hu* soothes the Liver and regulates *qi. Gan cao* harmonises all herbs.

## *Yin* Deficiency with Fire

Clinical manifestations: Depressed mood, irritability, sadness, loss of interest, loss of willpower, easily frightened, trance-like state, slow response and slow movements, hypochondriac distension and pain, abdominal distension and belching, loss of appetite, aching and cold lower back and knees, red complexion, night sweating, heat on the palms and soles, dry mouth and throat, red tongue with little coating, and string-like, thin and rapid pulse.

Treatment principle: Clear heat and soothe the Liver, enrich the Kidney and nourish *yin.*

Formula: Modified *Zi shui qin gan yin* 滋水清肝饮 加减.[1,2]

Herbs: *Shu di huang* 熟地黄, *dang gui* 当归, *shao yao* 芍药, *suan zao ren* 酸枣仁, *shan zhu yu* 山茱萸, *fu ling* 茯苓, *shan yao* 山药, *chai hu* 柴胡, *zhi zi* 栀子, *mu dan pi* 牡丹皮, and *ze xie* 泽泻.

Main action of herbs: *Shu di huang, shan yao,* and *shan zhu yu* enrich the Kidney and nourish *yin. Dang gui* tonifies *qi* and Blood. *Bai shao* nourishes Blood, replenishes *yin,* soothes the Liver and releases tension. *Fu ling* and *suan zao ren* tonify the Heart to calm the mind. *Chai hu* soothes the Liver and regulates *qi. Mu dan pi* and *zhi zi* cool Blood and clear heat. *Ze xie* drains dampness and purges heat.

## Deficiency of the Heart and Spleen

Clinical manifestations: Worry, paranoia, dizziness, lassitude, palpitations, timidity, insomnia, forgetfulness, loss of appetite, dull complexion, pale tongue with white and thin coating, and fine weak pulse.

Treatment principle: Tonify the Spleen and nourish the Heart, and tonify *qi* and Blood.

Formula: Modified *Gui pi tang* 归脾汤加减.[2,3]

Herbs: *Ren shen* 人参, *bai zhu* 白术, *huang qi* 黄芪, *dang gui* 当归, *fu ling* 茯苓, *yuan zhi* 远志, *suan zao ren* 酸枣仁, *mu xiang* 木香, *long yan rou* 龙眼肉, *gan cao* 甘草, *sheng jiang* 生姜, and *da zao* 大枣.

Main action of herbs: *Ren shen*, *bai zhu*, and *huang qi* tonify *qi* and the Spleen to generate Blood. *Dang gui* and *long yan rou* tonify *qi* and nourish the Heart. *Fu ling*, *suan zao ren*, and *yuan zhi* tonify the Heart to calm the mind. *Mu xiang* regulates *qi* and nourishes the Spleen. *Gan cao*, *sheng jiang*, and *da zao* harmonise the Spleen and the Stomach.

## Heart and Kidney *Yin* Deficiency

Clinical manifestations: Emotional instability, palpitations, forgetfulness, insomnia, dream-disturbed sleep, vexing heat in the chest, palms and soles, night sweats, thirst and dry throat, red tongue with little moisture and fine pulse.

Treatment principle: Tonify the Heart and Kidney *yin*.

Formula: Modified *Tian wang bu xin dan* combined with *Liu wei di huang wan* 天王补心丹合六味地黄丸加减.[3]

Herbs: *Di huang* 地黄, *shan yao* 山药, *shan zhu yu* 山茱萸, *tian dong* 天冬, *mai dong* 麦冬, *xuan shen* 玄参, *ren shen* 人参, *fu ling* 茯苓, *wu wei zi* 五味子, *dang gui* 当归, *bai zi ren* 柏子仁, *suan zao ren* 酸枣仁, *yuan zhi* 远志, *dan shen* 丹参, and *mu dan pi* 牡丹皮.

Main action of herbs: *Di huang*, *shan yao*, *shan zhu yu*, *tian dong*, *mai dong*, and *xuan shen* tonify the Heart and Kidney. *Ren shen*, *fu *ling, wu wei zi,* and *dang gui* tonify *qi* and Blood. *Bai zi ren, suan zao ren, yuan zhi,* and *dan shen* tonify the Heart to calm the mind. *Mu dan pi* cools the Blood and clears heat.

## Melancholy Disturbing the Mind

Clinical manifestations: Mental confusion, paranoia, easily frightened, sadness with crying, irritability, fatigue, overactive body movements, manic or delirious, pale tongue, and string-like pulse.

Treatment principle: Nourish the Heart to calm the mind, moisten and release tension using herbs with sweet properties.

Formula: Modified *Gan mai da zao tang* 甘麦大枣汤加减.[1-3]

Herbs: *Gan cao* 甘草, *xiao mai* 小麦, and *da zao* 大枣.

Main action of herbs: *Gan cao* releases tension with its sweet property. *Xiao mai* tonifies the Heart *qi. Da zao* tonifies Blood and replenishes the Spleen.

# Acupuncture Therapies

Acupuncture therapies have been documented since the *Huang Di Nei Jing* 黄帝内经 (written before AD 618). Acupuncture may alleviate the symptoms of depression and other physical symptoms. Excess syndromes should be treated with purging methods, while deficiency syndromes should be treated with tonifying methods. Commonly used acupuncture points are summarised below[1]:

Main acupoints: HT7 *Shenmen* 神门, PC6 *Neiguan* 内关, PC7 *Daling* 大陵, LR14 *Qimen* 期门, BL15 *Xinshu* 心俞, LI4 *Hegu* 合谷, and LR3 *Taichong* 太冲.

Main actions of the points[9]:

- HT7 *Shenmen* 神门 — calms the spirit, regulates and tonifies the Heart;

- PC6 *Neiguan* 内关 — unbinds the chest and regulates *qi,* regulates the Heart, calms the spirit, harmonises the Stomach and alleviates nausea and vomiting, clears heat, and opens the *yin* linking vessels;
- PC7 *Daling* 大陵 — clears heat from the Heart and calms the spirit, harmonises the Stomach and intestines, unbinds the chest, clears the nutritive level, and cools Blood;
- LR14 *Qimen* 期门 — spreads the Liver and regulates *qi,* invigorates Blood and disperses masses, and harmonises the Liver and Stomach;
- BL15 *Xinshu* 心俞 — tonifies and nourishes the Heart, regulates Heart *qi,* calms the spirit, unbinds the chest, resolves Blood stasis, and clears Heart fire;
- LI4 *Hegu* 合谷 — activates the channels, alleviates pain, and restores the *yang.*
- LR3 *Taichong* 太冲 — nourishes Liver Blood and Liver *yin,* and clears the head and eyes.

## Acupuncture Treatment based on Syndrome Differentiation

The Standards for the Diagnosis, Syndrome Differentiation and Evaluation of the Clinical Effect for Depression recommend using the main acupuncture points for depression (see list above). In addition, points specific for syndrome differentiation should be added.

**Liver *qi* stagnation**: Add LR2 *Xingjian* 行间 and BL18 *Ganshu* 肝俞.

**Liver *qi* stagnation and Spleen *qi* deficiency**: Add BL18 *Ganshu* 肝俞, BL20 *Pishu* 脾俞, and ST36 *Zusanli* 足三里.

**Liver-Gallbladder dampness-heat**: Add LR14 *Qimen* 期门, GB24 *Riyue* 日月, KI3 *Taixi* 太溪, and SP6 *Sanyinjiao* 三阴交.

***Yin* deficiency with fire syndrome**: Add BL23 *Shenshu* 肾俞, BL18 *Ganshu* 肝俞, and KI3 *Taixi* 太溪.

**Melancholy disturbing the mind**: Add GV20 *Baihui* 百会, HT5 *Tongli* 通里, and GB24 *Riyue* 日月.

# Other Management Strategies

## Diet Therapy

The Guideline for Diagnosis and Treatment of Common Internal Diseases in Chinese Medicine-Symptoms of Modern Medicine recommends diet therapy for treating depression.[1] Liver *qi* stagnation and Spleen *qi* deficiency can be treated with *Mei gui ju hua* porridge 玫瑰菊花粥; ingredients include: *Mei gui hua* 玫瑰花, *ju hua* 菊花, and glutinous rice 糯米. The main actions of the porridge are to regulate *qi*, soothe the Liver and tonify the Spleen. People with *yin* deficiency and fire can be given *Long mu lian zi* soup 龙牡莲子羹; ingredients include: *Long gu* 龙骨, *mu li* 牡蛎, *zhi mu* 知母, *lian zi* 莲子, and sugar. The soup is used to calm the mind, enrich *yin* and purge fire.

Melancholy disturbing the mind can be treated with *Bai he suan zao ren* porridge 百合酸枣仁粥. Ingredients include: *Bai he* 百合, *suan zao ren* 酸枣仁, and rice. The main actions of the porridge include nourishing *yin* and tonifying Blood to calm the mind. *Bai he* porridge 百合粥 can also be used for melancholy disturbing the mind. Ingredients include: *Bai he* 百合, rice, and sugar. The main actions include tonifying *yin* and harmonising the middle, and tonifying the Heart to calm the mind.

# References

1. 中华中医药学会. (2008) 中医内科常见病诊疗指南•中医疾病部分. 北京: 中国中医药出版社.
2. 中国中医科学院. (2011) 中医循证临床实践指南. 中医内科. 北京: 中国中医药出版社.
3. 周仲瑛. (2007) 中医内科学（普通高等教育"十二五"国家级规划教材）. 北京:中国中医药出版社.
4. 董湘玉. (2007) 中医心理学（卫生部"十一五"规划教材;全国高等医药教材建设研究会划教材. 北京: 人民卫生出版社.
5. 黄培新,黄燕. (2013) 神经科专病中医临床诊治（第三版）. 北京: 人民卫生出版社.
6. 赵永厚, 蔡定芳. (2009) 中医神志病学. 上海: 上海中医药大学出版社.

7.  唐启盛. (2012) 抑郁障碍中西医基础与临床. 北京: 人民卫生出版社.

8.  中华医学会精神医学分会. (2015) 中国抑郁障碍防治指南（第二版）. 北京: 中华医学电子音像出版社.

9.  Deadman P, Baker K and Al-Khafaji M. (2007) A Manual of Acupuncture. 2nd ed. Journal of Chinese Medicine Publications.

# 3

# Classical Chinese Medicine Literature

## OVERVIEW

Classical Chinese texts record the traditional use of Chinese medicine. The classical texts informed clinical practice throughout the ancient period and continue to be used today. This chapter includes findings from a search of the classical Chinese medicine literature from AD 206 to 1949. A total of 4,806 citations were found and 319 described depression. Of the Chinese medicine therapies, herbal formulae were most commonly used for depression.

## Introduction

Written records of the professional practice of Chinese medicine (CM) date back to the Spring and Autumn (770–476 BC) and Warring states (474–221 BC) periods. In these passages, concepts such as *yin* and *yang* are evident, and therapeutic methods included the use of herbal decoctions and acupuncture.[1] The word "depression" is found in medical books as old as the *Huang Di Nei Jing* 黄帝内经 (written before AD 618); related terms such as sad, unhappy, or worry can also be found. *Huang Di Nei Jing* also described the negative effects of these emotions on one's well being. Information on depression diagnosis and treatment increased in volume and detail with time, with the peak period being the Ming and Qing dynasties, where depression is described in a similar way as in modern literature. In order to obtain a sample of the classical and pre-modern medical literature on depression we conducted electronic searches of the *Zhong Hua Yi Dian* 中华医典 (ZHYD), a CD of more than 1,000 medical books.[2] This collection is the largest currently available and is representative of other large collections of the classical and pre-modern CM literature.[3,4]

## Search Terms

Unipolar depression and major depressive disorder are modern disease names and cannot be used to search for classical literature in the ZHYD. However, CM disease terminologies include various traditional disease names of potential relevance to depression. For example, *yu* 郁 and *yu bing* 郁病 can refer to "depression" and "depressive disease". In addition, *you* 忧 and *bei* 悲 are terms associated with "sadness". There are also CM diseases that are not directly called "depression" but present with depressive symptoms. For instance, *zang zao* 脏躁, a disease caused by *yin* deficiency of the *zang* organs, presents with an inability to concentrate, sadness, a tendency to cry, unstable mood, and restlessness.

To select search terms to use in the ZHYD, a number of dictionaries, monographs, medical nomenclatures and textbooks specific for a CM understanding of depression, as well as experts, were consulted.[5–11] Using the selected search terms, the ZHYD was then searched and the citations were screened for relevance. Selected search terms most relevant to depression were categorised into four groups: 1) *Yu* 郁 (depression) and its synonyms; 2) Depressive symptomatic terms such as sadness and its synonyms, fatigue, and loss of ambition; 3) Chinese medicine disease terms that present with depressive disorder symptoms; and 4) Suicide and its synonyms.

## Search Procedure and Data Coding

Each term was entered into the ZHYD search fields and the search results were downloaded to excel spread sheets. A "citation" was defined as a distinct passage of text referring to one or more of the search terms. Codes were allocated for types of citations, books, and the dynasties in which they were written according to the procedures described in May *et al.,* 2014.[4] Books written after 1949 were excluded.

# Data Analysis Procedure

The number of hits identified by each search term was calculated by summing the results of the searches. After removing duplicates, exclusion criteria were then applied to remove citations which were considered not related to depression (i.e. not relevant). Duplicates and citations related to children were removed from the dataset. To exclude other types of depression, we removed citations that were relevant to psychiatric disorders (i.e. 癲狂 *dian kuang*, madness, visual and auditory hallucinations) and depression caused by physical diseases.

All relevant citations were reviewed to identify the best descriptions of depression and its aetiology or pathogenesis. Citations which did not include treatment were excluded from further analysis. The final dataset includes citations considered to potentially refer to unipolar depression, which described CM treatments (Chinese herbal medicine [CHM], acupuncture and related therapies, or other CM therapies). When a citation referred to multiple treatments, each treatment was considered as a separate citation for calculation of formulae, herbs, or acupuncture points. Citations which were pharmacopeia-type entries were reviewed for eligibility. Pharmacopeia entries which mentioned the name of the condition, but did not include a detailed description of the condition or information about treatment, were excluded from further analysis. Pharmacopeia entries which included a description of the condition, with or without reference to other herbs, were included. Single acupuncture points were reviewed in a similar manner.

Included citations were grouped according to the CM intervention for further analysis. An additional screening process was performed to identify citations considered "most likely" to be depression. A judgment of "most likely" was made when a citation described at least one of the main symptoms of "depressed mood" or "loss of interest", plus two or more of the following symptoms: change in appetite or sleep, psychomotor agitation, fatigue, feeling of worthlessness or excessive or inappropriate guilt, diminished ability to think or concentrate, suicidal thoughts, irritability, and tension or anxiety. Data are presented for the frequencies of identified formulae, herbs and acupuncture points for citations related to depression.

## Search Results

In total, 4,806 citations were found using the search terms outlined in Table 3.1. The citations were identified from 649 books, with the highest number of citations coming from *Ben Cao Gang Mu* 本草纲目 (AD 1578) (22 citations, 6.5%). The earliest book that mentioned depression was the *Huang Di Nei Jing* 黄帝内经 (AD 618), and the

**Table 3.1. Hit Frequency by Search Term**

| Pinyin | Chinese Characters | Hit Frequency (n, %) |
|---|---|---|
| *You si* | 忧思 | 925 (19.3) |
| *You lv* | 忧虑 | 825 (17.2) |
| *Shi zhi* | 失志 | 447 (9.3) |
| *Bai he bing* | 百合病 | 416 (8.7) |
| *Bei shang* | 悲伤 | 374 (7.8) |
| *Yu* | 郁 | 321 (6.7) |
| *Zi yi* | 自缢 | 254 (5.3) |
| *Mei he qi* | 梅核气 | 246 (5.1) |
| *Bei* | 悲 | 195 (4.1) |
| *Yu zheng* | 郁证 | 180 (3.8) |
| *Yu zheng* | 郁症 | 144 (3.0) |
| *Zi jin* | 自尽 | 103 (2.1) |
| *Yu bing* | 郁病 | 80 (1.7) |
| *Ben tun qi* | 奔豚气 | 72 (1.5) |
| *Zang zao* | 脏躁 | 66 (1.4) |
| *You* | 忧 | 47 (1.0) |
| *Zi sha* | 自杀 | 45 (0.9) |
| *Zi wen* | 自刎 | 38 (0.8) |
| *Bei die* | 卑惵 | 23 (0.5) |
| *Shen tui* | 神颓 | 5 (0.1) |

most recent book was the *Ben Cao Jian Yao Fang* 本草简要方 (AD 1938). The majority of citations came from the Qing dynasty (1645–1911 AD) (2,216 citations, 46.1%), followed by the Ming dynasty (1369–1644 AD) (1,291 citations, 26.9%).

The term *you si* 忧思 (sadness with overthinking) found the most citations (925) and *you lv* 忧虑 (sadness with excessive worry) found the second largest number of citations (825). Terms directly related to depression symptoms such as *shi zhi* 失志, *bai he bing* 百合病, and *bei shang* 悲伤 also found high numbers of citations. Table 3.1 includes the number and proportion of citations obtained by each search term. Search terms *bei die* 卑慄 and *shen tui* 神颓 produced the smallest number of citations. Some citations were identified by more than one search term, therefore the total percentage may exceed 100.

After reviewing all 4,806 citations, 319 related to depression and are included for further analysis. Of these, 256 citations were judged to be 'most likely' related to depression. A total of 290 citations described depressed mood, 13 citations did not describe depressed mood, 16 citations mentioned depression, or depressive symptoms, but did not specify depressed mood, 103 citations clearly stated loss of interest, 206 citations did not specify loss of interest, and 10 citations had no description of loss of interest. Citations that did not clearly state depressed mood or loss of interest, and citations that had a CM diagnosis of *bei die*, *yu bing*, *yu zheng*, or *zang zao*, but did not specify these two symptoms, those were excluded for further analysis. More than one-third (36%) of citations were specific to women, in which 25 citations were postpartum specific, having a syndrome of *zang zao* 脏躁.

## Frequency of Treatment Citations by Dynasty

Books from the Ming and Qing dynasties accounted for the largest proportion of citations (84.6%).[1-3] This indicates that knowledge on the disease was at its peak during these times. Table 3.2 presents the distribution of citations with treatment information by dynasty. Several key books from the Qing and Ming dynasties included: *Ji Yin Gang Mu* 济阴纲目 (AD 1620), *Yi Xue Ru Men* 医学入门 (AD 1575),

Table 3.2.   Dynastic Distribution of Treatment Citations

| Dynasty | No. of Treatment Citations |
|---|---|
| Before Tang Dynasty (before 618) | 2 |
| Tang and 5 Dynasties (618–960) | 1 |
| Song and Jin Dynasties (961–1271) | 5 |
| Yuan Dynasty (1272–1368) | 4 |
| Ming Dynasty (1369–1644) | 122 |
| Qing Dynasty (1645–1911) | 148 |
| Ming Guo/Republic of China (1912–1949) | 7 |
| Japanese literature (before 1949) | 8 |
| **Total** | **319** |

*Jing Yue Quan Shu* 景岳全书 (AD 1624), *Za Bing Yuan Liu Xi Zhu* 杂病源流犀烛 (AD 1773), *Bu Ju Ji* 不居集 (AD 1739), and *Lei Zheng Zhi Cai* 类证治裁 (AD 1839).

## Definitions of the Condition and Aetiology

Several citations included detailed information on the aetiology and pathogenesis of depression. *Ye Tianshi* in the Qing dynasty wrote in *Lin Zheng Zhi Nan Yi An* 临证指南医案 (AD 1746) "Depression is often caused by emotional disturbances. For example, worry will damage the Spleen and anger damages the Liver. Its root cause is the Heart, disturbed by emotional upset and leading to *Yu* stagnation. In turn causing *qi* stagnation, which overtime becomes Heat and consumes *Jing* fluids, disturbing the dispersing and distributing mechanism. Short-term affecting the *qi* level, long-term effecting the Blood level, eventually leading to depression." 清•叶天士《临证指南医案•郁》: "七情之郁居多, 如思伤脾, 怒伤肝之类是也, 其原总由于心, 因情感不遂, 则郁而成病矣。皆因郁则气滞, 气滞久则必化热, 热郁则津液耗而不流, 升降之机失度, 初伤气分, 久延血分, 延及郁劳沉病".

In *Gu Jin Yi Tong* (AD 1556) by *Xu Chunpu* in the Ming dynasty, it described that "depression is caused by the disturbance of the seven emotions, leading to stagnation, signs and symptoms are diverse overtime." 明·徐春甫《古今医统》: 曰"郁为七情不舒,遂成郁结,既郁之久, 变病多端".

The effect of negative emotions on *zang fu* organs is described in *Ling Shu* (AD 221) "Sadness and worry will damage the Heart, then lead to imbalance of the *zang fu* organs." 《灵枢·口问》云: "悲哀愁忧则心动, 心动则五脏六腑皆摇". A similar theory is also described in *Su Wen* (AD 221) "Worry and overthinking will damage the Heart." 《素问·本病论》: "人忧愁思虑即伤心".

In *Wan Bing Hui Chun* (AD 1587) by *Gong Yanting* in the Ming dynasty, *mei he* is described to be "mainly caused by emotional upsets leading to depression or getting upset while eating leading to stagnation. It is more common in women. Treatment should focus on removing stagnation, regulating *qi*, clearing the Lungs and removing phlegm." 明·龚延庭《万病回春》: "梅核为病, 大抵因七情之气郁结而成, 或因饮食之时触犯恼怒, 遂成此症, 惟妇人女子患此最多. 治宜开郁顺气, 利隔化痰清肺为主".

# Chinese Herbal Medicine

Chinese herbal formulae were the most common therapies for depression, accounting for 297 (93.1%) of cited treatments. Some formulae did not have a name and just included the herbal ingredients. Eight citations combined oral formulae with external wash therapy. Table 3.3 includes the most frequent formulae found in depression citations.

## Most Frequent Formulae in Depression Citations

In the depression citations, modified *Gan mai da zao tang* 甘麦大枣汤 and *Gui pi tang* 归脾汤 were the most frequently used treatments. There were 20 citations that did not provide a formula name, but five citations had the same herb ingredients as *Gan mai da zao tang* 甘麦大枣汤.

*Gan mai da zao tang* 甘麦大枣汤 first appeared in the book *Jin Gui Yao Lue* 金匮要略 (AD 206) and is still commonly used in contemporary clinical practice. This simple formula nourishes the Heart and calms the mind, and treats the CM disease *zang zao*. In females and

**Table 3.3.  Most Frequent Formulae in Depression Citations**

| Formula Name | Herb Ingredients | No. of Citations (n) |
|---|---|---|
| Gan mai da zao tang 甘麦大枣汤 | Gan cao 甘草, xiao mai 小麦, and da zao 大枣 | 63 |
| Gui pi tang/wan 归脾汤/丸 | Bai zhu 白术, dang gui 当归, fu ling 茯苓, huang qi 黄芪, long yan rou 龙眼肉, yuan zhi 远志, suan zao ren 酸枣仁, mu xiang 木香, gan cao 甘草, and ren shen 人参 | 29 |
| Qi fu yin 七福饮 | Ren shen 人参, shu di huang 熟地黄, dang gui 当归, bai zhu 白术, gan cao甘草, suan zao ren 酸枣仁, and yuan zhi 远志 | 8 |
| Qi qi tang 七气汤 | Ren shen 人参, gan cao 甘草, rou gui 肉桂, and ban xia 半夏 | 7 |
| Ren shen yang rong tang 人参养荣汤 | Ren shen 人参, bai zhu 白术, huang qi 黄芪, gan cao 甘草, chen pi 陈皮, rou gui 肉桂, dang gui 当归, shu di huang 熟地黄, wu wei zi 五味子, fu ling 茯苓, yuan zhi 远志, and shao yao 芍药 | 7 |
| Zi su zi tang 紫苏子汤 | Zi su zi 紫苏子, da fu pi 大腹皮, cao guo 草果, ban xia 半夏, hou po 厚朴, mu xiang 木香, chen pi 陈皮, mu tong 木通, bai zhu 白术, zhi shi 枳实, ren shen 人参, and gan cao 甘草 | 7 |
| Xiao yan san 逍遥散 | Chai hu 柴胡, dang gui 当归, shao yao 芍药, bai zhu 白术, fu ling 茯苓, sheng jiang 生姜, bo he 薄荷, and gan cao 甘草 | 6 |
| Dan zhu ru tang 淡竹茹汤 | Mai dong 麦冬, xiao mai 小麦, ban xia 半夏, ren shen 人参, fu ling 茯苓, gan cao 甘草, sheng jiang 生姜, da zao 大枣, and dan zhu ru 淡竹茹 | 6 |
|  | Dan zhu ru 淡竹茹, mai dong 麦冬, gan cao 甘草, xiao mai 小麦, sheng jiang 生姜, and da zao 大枣 | 5 |
| Sheng chai jun zi tang 升柴四君子汤 | Ren shen 人参, bai zhu 白术, fu ling 茯苓, gan cao 甘草, chai hu 柴胡, shan zhi zi 山栀子, and sheng ma 升麻 | 5 |

**Table 3.3.** (*Continued*)

| Formula Name | Herb Ingredients | No. of Citations (n) |
|---|---|---|
| Wen dan tang 温胆汤 | Bai xia半夏, dan zhu ru 淡竹茹, zhi shi 枳实, chen pi 陈皮, gan cao 甘草, and fu ling 茯苓 | 5 |
| Chen xiang jiang qi tang 沉香降气汤 | Xiang fu 香附, chen xiang 沉香, sha ren 砂仁, and gan cao 甘草 | 4 |
| Bai he di huang tang 百合地黄汤 | Bai he 百合, and sheng di huang 生地黄 | 4 |
| Er chen tang 二陈汤 | Chen pi 陈皮, ban xia 半夏, fu ling 茯苓, bai zhu 白术, cang zhu 苍术, sha ren 砂仁, shan yao 山药, che qian zi车前子, mu tong 木通, hou po 厚朴, and gan cao 甘草 | 4 |
|  | Ban xia 半夏, ju hong 橘红, fu ling 茯苓, gan cao 甘草, shao yao 芍药, dang gui 当归, wu yao 乌药, qin pi 青皮, zhi ke 枳壳, xiang fu 香附, hou po 厚朴, and zi su ye 紫苏叶 | 1 |
| Bu zhong yi qi tang 补中益气汤 | Huang qi 黄芪, gan cao 甘草, ren shen 人参, dang gui 当归, chen pi 陈皮, sheng ma 升麻, chai hu 柴胡, and bai zhu 白术 | 3 |

*Note*: The use of some herbs such as *mu xiang* 木香 may be restricted in some countries; readers are advised to comply with relevant regulations.

postpartum, the majority used *Gan mai da zao tang* 甘麦大枣汤 as the treatment. In *Jin Gui* it is said that "woman with *zang zao* feel sad and have a tendency to cry with no apparent cause, frequent yawning, and should be treated with *Gan mai da zao tang* (《金匮》有一证云: 妇人脏躁悲伤欲哭, 象如神灵所作, 数欠伸者, 宜甘麦大枣汤).

## Most Frequent Herbs in Depression Citations

There were 151 herbs used in the herbal formulae, the most frequent herb was *gan cao* 甘草, being the chief herb in *Gan mai da zao tang* 甘麦大枣汤 and also a harmonising herb. Table 3.4 includes the most frequent herbs found in depression citations.

**Table 3.4.    Most Frequent Herbs in Depression Citations**

| Herb Name | Scientific Name | No. of Citations (n) |
|---|---|---|
| Gan cao/zhi gan cao 甘草 (炙) | *Glycyrrhiza spp.* | 238 (232/6) |
| Ren shen 人参 | *Panax ginseng* C.A. Mey | 123 |
| Fu ling/fu shen 茯苓 (茯神) | *Porias cocos (Schw.)* Wolf | 119 (99/20) |
| Bai zhu 白术 | *Atractylodes macrocephala Koidz* | 98 |
| Dang gui 当归 | *Angelica sinensis* (Oliv.) Diels | 93 |
| Da zao 大枣 | *Ziziphus jujube* Mill. | 92 |
| Xiao mai 小麦 | *Triticum aestivum* L. | 79 |
| Yuan zhi 远志 | *Polygala tenuifolia* Willd. var. sibirica L. | 68 |
| Mu xiang 木香 | Aucklandia lappa Decne. | 62 |
| Suan zao ren 酸枣仁 | *Ziziphus jujuba* Mill. var. *spinosa* (Bunge) Hu ex H. F. Chou | 58 |
| Jiang/sheng jiang/gan jiang 姜(生姜/干姜) | *Zingiber officinale* Rosc. | 51 (8/34/9) |
| Chen pi 陈皮 | *Citrus reticulata* Blanco | 50 |
| Di huang 地黄 | *Rehmannia glutinosa* Libosch. | 47 |
| Shao yao 芍药 | *Paeonia lactiflora* Pall. | 40 |
| Ban xia 半夏 | *Pinellia ternata* (Thunb.) Breit. | 36 |
| Long yan rou 龙眼肉 | *Dimocarpus longan* Lour. | 36 |
| Rou gui/gui zhi 肉桂/桂枝 | *Cinnamomum cassia* Presl | 37 (33/4) |
| Chai hu 柴胡 | *Bupleurum chinense DC.* var. *scorzonerifolium Willd.* | 33 |
| Zhi shi 枳实 | *Citrus aurantium* L. var. *sinensis* Osbeck | 28 |
| Mai dong 麦冬 | *Ophiopogon japonicus* (L.f) Ker-Gawl. | 27 |
| Shan zhi zi 山栀子 | *Gardenia jasminoides* Ellis | 23 |

*Note*: The use of some herbs such as *mu xiang* 木香 may be restricted in some countries; readers are advised to comply with relevant regulations.

## Herbal Wash

Herbal medicine was used as external therapy to treat conditions caused by depression, such as *mei he qi* 梅核气 (feeling of something stuck in the throat) and melasma. One citation, from the book *Li Yue Pian Wen* by *Wu Shangxian* in the Qing dynasty, described using herbs as an external wipe for the treatment of *mei he qi* 梅核气. It stated that "Women with irregular menstruation due to stagnation in the meridians, also present with *mei he qi* 梅核气, where it feels like something is stuck in the throat but cannot be swallowed nor expelled, caused by *qi* and phlegm stagnation. Use *zi su, hou po, ban xia, chi fu ling, cang zhu, zhi shi, chen pi, tian nan xing, xiang fu, sha ren, shen qu, qin pi, zhi zi, bing lang, yi zhi ren, huang lian, sheng jiang* and *xing ren*, crush together and wipe the neck area". 【理瀹骈文】妇人经水不调壅塞经络亦令喉肿宜通经又有梅核气喉中如有物吞不入吐不出气郁痰结也妇人为多紫苏厚朴半夏赤苓苍术枳实陈皮南星香附砂仁神曲青皮栀子槟榔益智仁黄连生姜各一钱杏仁捣丸擦.

Another citation described the use of herbal wash for melasma caused by worry and depression with the focus primarily on the skin problem. In *Wai Ke Xin Fa Yao Jue* (AD 1742), *Qi Hongyuan* wrote: "Melasma, like dirt on the face, can be the size of lotus seed or red bean, caused by worry and depression, can be treated by *Yu rong san*". 【外科心法要诀】如尘久炱暗，原于忧思抑郁成，大如莲子小赤豆, 玉容久洗自然平.

## Combination Therapies

There were 10 citations combining oral herbal medicine and other therapies. One citation from the book *Bian Que Xin Shu* combined herbal formulae and moxibustion for depressive symptoms, it stated that "when one reaches middle-age, his constitution will weaken, Heart-Blood may be consumed by overthinking, melancholy, or greed, until *Jing qi* is depleted and results in death. Treat with moxibustion on CV4 *Guanyuan* 关元 plus CHM formula *Yan shou dan".*【扁鹊心书.神痴病】凡人至中年, 天数自然虚衰, 或加妄想忧思, 或为功名失志, 以致心血大耗, 痴醉不治, 渐至精气耗尽而死, 当灸关元穴三百壮, 服延寿丹一斤.

Eight citations combined oral formulae with external wash therapy. All eight citations used the same herbs for external therapy for vaginal sores possibly caused by depression: *Jing jie* 荆芥, *zhi ke* 枳壳, *he zi* 诃子, and *wu bei zi* 五倍子. *Wai Ke Xin Fa Yao Jue* wrote "female genital sores caused by excessive sadness and overthinking, should use *Xiao yao san* or *Gui pi tang* modified, when postpartum, use *Bu zhong yi qi tang* modified, use *jing jie, zhi ke, he zi, wen ge* as external wash".【外科心法要诀.妇人阴疮】由忧思太过所致, 宜逍遥散或归脾汤俱加柴胡、栀子、白芍、丹皮服之; 由产后得者, 补中益气汤加五味子、醋炒白芍服之, 外俱用荆芥、枳壳、诃子、文蛤, 大剂煎汤熏洗.

One citation combined oral herbal formula with an acupuncture technique. It described the use of a small needle to let a small amount of blood out, the citation was used to treat obstruction in the throat with pharyngitis which is possibly caused by depression. *Hou Ke Ji Ye* wrote "wind-heat type throat obstruction with pharyngitis caused by worrying, excessive fatigue or talking in windy conditions, leading to wind attacking the Lung meridian, the utmost important treatment is expelling the phlegm. For pharyngitis, use a small needle to let some blood out and follow by oral herbal formula *Bing pian san".*【喉科集腋.喉痹】风热喉痹由于忧思劳碌太过或对风言语风入肺经作痰务多去痰为要其色鲜红久而紫赤急用小刀刺破血微出火已泻矣再服煎剂吹冰片散.

## Acupuncture and Related Therapies

Acupuncture and moxibustion citations for depression were scarce; it was only described in eight citations (acupuncture 5, moxibustion 3). Four citations were from before the Tang dynasty and the other four were spread out in various dynasties.

In the *Huang Di Nei Jing Tai Su* (AD 616), it states that "those who are sad can be treated from the *jue yin* meridian, tonify or reduce depending on the disease condition". 【黄帝内经太素】悲者取之厥阴, 视有余不足. Acupuncture points include PC7 *Daling* 大陵, PC5 *Jianshi* 间使, PC6 *Neiguan* 内关, KI6 *Zhaohai* 照海, and BL15 *Xinshu* 心腧. In *Zhen Jiu Jia Yi Jing* (AD 282), *Yang Shangshan* (Sui dynasty) described "heartache, feeling sorrow, *qi* upsurge, emptiness in the Heart, feeling no interest and edgy, use PC7 *Daling* and PC5 *Jianshi*; feeling no interest and frightened, feeling sad, use PC6 *Nei guan*". 【针灸甲乙经】心痛善悲, 厥逆, 悬心如饥之状 (饿的时候心挂着的感觉), 心淡淡而惊 (淡漠又害怕慌张), 大陵及间使主之. 心淡淡而善惊恐 (淡漠又容易受惊吓), 心悲, 内关主之. Another citation from this book stated: "Feeling edgy, unhappy and depressed, feeling down, no sweating, dark complexion, no appetite, use KI6 *Zhao hai*." 【针灸甲乙经】惊, 善悲不乐, 如堕坠 (feel so down), 汗不出, 面尘黑, 病饮不欲食, 照海主之.

Out of the three citations describing moxibustion treatment for depression, only one citation gave details on the point which is the ear lobe 耳垂. *Hou Ke Jia Xun* by *Diao Buzhong* (Qing dynasty) stated: "To treat a lump under the skin between the ear and the neck the size of a plum stone, that is caused by depression with worry and sadness, plus external pathogens in the *tai yang* meridian, or anger affecting the Liver that damages the tendons, worry affecting the Spleen that cause muscles to swell up. In the beginning it is swollen and painful, over time it becomes rotten and hard to heal. In extreme cases it causes teeth to fall out and rotten gums, use moxibustion on *Er chui* (ear lobe)." 【喉科家训】治忧思郁虑, 邪毒交乘结聚太阳经络, 或恼怒伤肝致筋骨紧急, 思虑伤脾致肌肉结肿,膏粱厚味致脓名臭秽, 其状於耳项皮肤间隐隐有核渐如桃李便觉肿痛,初则坚硬不消, 久则延烂难愈, 甚致齿牙堕落, 牙床腐秽.....以陈艾灸耳垂. Another moxibustion citation from *Bian Que Xin Shu* by *Dou Cai* in the year 1146 stated: "For those who are experiencing loss of confidence and loss of interest, firstly ought to change their temperament, have a drink to relax and use moxibustion to treat." 【扁鹊心书】失志不遂之病, 非排遣性情不可, 以灸法操其要, 醉酒陶其情, 此法妙极.

## Discussion

Books from the Ming and Qing dynasties accounted for the largest proportion of the depression citations, indicating knowledge of the disease and its treatment was at its peak during these times. The majority of citations described oral herbal formulae and there were very few acupuncture and moxibustion citations. The reason is unknown; however, these treatment types may have been unpopular for treating depression and herbal medicine produced a superior effect.

Each citation was judged to be related to depression based on symptom presentation: Main symptoms, depressed mood or loss of interest; and associated symptoms: Change in appetite or sleep, psychomotor agitation, fatigue, feeling of worthlessness, excessive or inappropriate guilt, diminished ability to think or concentrate, thoughts of death, irritability, tension or anxiety. We found that the most common main symptom was depressed mood and the most common associated symptoms were tension and anxiety. This finding is in line with the contemporary understanding of depression, where tension or anxiety correlates with depression.

In the Ming dynasty in the year 1602, *Zheng zhi zhun shen* 证治准绳, written by *Wang Kentang* described "one with loss of interest and loss of confidence, because they cannot achieve what they desire or regrets and blames themselves for the past, has no appetite, feels guilty, prefers to stay in dark rooms or behind doors, avoids contact with people, this is called *bei die* disease, due to Blood deficiency."【证治准绳】有失志者, 由所求不遂, 或过误自咎, 懊恨嗟叹不已, 独语书空, 若有所失……有痞塞不饮食, 心中常有所歉, 爱处暗地, 或倚门后, 见人则惊避, 似失志状, 此为卑愫之病, 以血不足故耳. This citation clearly described the CM aetiology and diagnosis of *bei die* disease, and its symptoms, which are comparable to depression.

*Za Bing Guang Yao* by the Japanese author *Dan Bo Yuan Jian* in the year 1853 wrote: "Stagnation in the Spleen, no appetite for six months, or feverish at noon that subsides in the late evening (5–9 pm), or feels irritable, thirsty, nausea, or feels sleepy but cannot fall asleep, always sits in the corner and likes dark places, women has scanty menses, men has urinary incontinence. This is all caused by worry and sadness leading to *qi* deficiency. Treat using *Wen dan tang* or *Er chen tang* plus *ren shen, bai zhu* and *fu ling*". 【杂病广要】有郁结在脾, 半年不食, 或午后发热, 酉戌时退, 或烦闷作渴虽呕, 或困卧如痴, 向里坐, 亦喜向暗处, 妇人经水极少, 男子小便点滴, 皆忧思气结, 治宜温胆汤, 或二陈汤加参、术、红花. This citation describes the cause, symptoms and treatments for depression.

In *Yang Yi Da Quan* 疡医大全, published in the Qing dynasty in the year 1760, Doctor *Gu Shicheng* wrote: "For *qi* stagnation syndrome, personal and social instability, loss of interest in fame and fortune, feeling depressed and irritable, no appetite, ill-looking complexion and lean body stature, chest fullness, *Jiao gan dan* is an effective treatment, when received well, it can clear Heart fire and nourish the Kidney water." 【疡医大全】交感丹治诸气郁滞, 一切公私拂情, 名利失志, 抑郁烦恼, 七情所伤, 不思饮食, 面黄形羸, 胸膈痞闷诸证神效, 大能升降水火.

## Classical Literature in Perspective

Unipolar depression and major depressive disorder are modern terms and cannot be used to identify information in classical CM literature. However, terms that relate to depression have been described in the classical texts as early as the *Huang Di Nei Jing* 黄帝内经. A large number of classical literature citations relate to depression and its accompanied symptoms. In ancient China, CM doctors treated depression based on aetiology, as well as CM syndromes such as *qi* and phlegm stagnation or *qi* deficiency. Depression was often related to CM disease diagnosis of *bei die* 卑慄, *mei he qi* 梅核气, *zang zao* 脏燥, *bai he bing* 百合病, *and ben tun qi* 奔豚气. Furthermore, depression was often described as a disease and not according to symptoms like the modern guidelines for disease classification. Depression in women and postpartum was commonly found, this is interesting as modern data indicate that women experience depression more than men.

The most common formulae and herbs identified in the classical literature are still widely used today, such as *Gan mai da zao tang* 甘麦大枣汤 and *Gui pi tang* 归脾汤. These formulae are recommended in the modern clinical guidelines for depression. *Gan mai da zao tang* 甘麦大枣汤 was commonly used in women with *zang zao* 脏燥 disease. The main categories of herbs used for depression include disperse Liver *qi* and harmonise the Stomach, tonify Spleen and regulate *qi*, calm the mind and nourish the Heart, nourish *yin* and remove irritability and warm the *yang* and tonify *qi*. *Gan cao* 甘草was the most commonly cited herb, likely due to its inclusion as a harmonising herb in many formulae, including the key formula *Gan mai da zao tang* 甘麦大枣汤. Other commonly cited herbs included *fu ling* 茯苓, *ren shen* 人参, *bai zhu* 白术, and *dang gui* 当归.

Contemporary depression treatment often includes acupuncture. However, it was only found in a few classical citations. In the studies that did use acupuncture, points included PC7 *Daling* 大陵, PC5 *Jianshi* 间使, PC6 *Neiguan* 内关, KI3 *Zhaohai* 照海, and BL15 *Xinshu* 心腧.

# References

1. Needham J, Lu GD, and Sivin N. (2000) Science and civilisation in China, Vol 5, Pt VI: Medicine. Cambridge: Cambridge University Press.
2. Hu R. (ed.) (2000) Zhong Hua Yi Dian "Encyclopaedia of Traditional Chinese Medicine". 4th ed., Changsha: Hunan Electronic and Audio-Visual Publishing House, 2000.
3. May BH, Lu CJ, and Xue CCL. (2012) Collections of traditional Chinese medical literature as resources for systematic searches, *J Altern Complement Med* **18**(12): 1101–1107.
4. May BH, Lu YB, Lu CJ, *et al.* (2013) Systematic assessment of the representativeness of published collections of the traditional literature on Chinese Medicine. *J Altern Complement Med* **19**(5): 403–409.
5. 中华中医药学会. (2008) 中医内科常见病诊疗指南•中医疾病部分. 北京: 中国中医药出版社.
6. 中国中医科学院. (2011) 中医循证临床实践指南. 中医内科. 北京: 中国中医药出版社.
7. 周仲瑛. (2007) 中医内科学（普通高等教育"十二五"国家级规划教材）. 北京: 中国中医药出版社.

8. 董湘玉. (2007) 中医心理学（卫生部"十一五"规划教材;全国高等医药教材建设研究会划教材. 北京: 人民卫生出版社.
9. 黄培新, 黄燕. (2013) 神经科专病中医临床诊治（第三版). 北京: 人民卫生出版社.
10. 赵永厚, 蔡定芳. (2009) 中医神志病学. 上海: 上海中医药大学出版社.
11. 唐启盛. (2012) 抑郁障碍中西医基础与临床. 北京: 人民卫生出版社.

# 4

# Methods for Evaluating Clinical Evidence

### OVERVIEW

This chapter describes the methods used to identify and evaluate a range of Chinese medicine interventions for depression in clinical studies. Studies identified through a comprehensive search were assessed against eligibility criteria. A review of the methodological quality of the studies was undertaken using standardised methods. Results from included studies were evaluated to provide an estimate of the effects of a range of Chinese medicine therapies.

## Introduction

The use of Chinese medicine (CM) for depression has been well described in contemporary literature. Several systematic reviews have been conducted to evaluate the efficacy and safety of CM treatments for depression. These have included eight reviews of Chinese herbal medicines (CHMs), and six reviews of acupuncture.

Chinese medicine interventions for depression in clinical studies have been examined. Interventions have been categorised as follows:

- Chinese herbal medicine (Chapter 5);
- Acupuncture and related therapies (Chapter 7);
- Other CM therapies (Chapter 8);
- Combination CM therapies (Chapter 9).

References to clinical trials were obtained and assessed by an expert group. Randomised controlled trials (RCTs), non-randomised controlled clinical trials (CCTs) and non-controlled studies were evaluated in detail. Controlled trials were evaluated using the same

**Table 4.1. Chinese Medicine Interventions Included in Clinical Evidence Evaluation**

| Category | Intervention |
| --- | --- |
| Chinese herbal medicines | Oral Chinese herbal medicine |
| Acupuncture and related therapies | Acupuncture, ear acupuncture, electroacupuncture, laser acupuncture, and scalp acupuncture therapy |
| Other Chinese medicine therapies | *Tuina* 推拿 (Chinese massage) and cupping |
| Combination Chinese medicine | Combination therapies are defined as two or more Chinese medicine interventions from different categories administered together. They included Chinese herbal medicines and acupuncture; acupuncture and moxibustion; acupuncture and cupping; acupuncture and *tuina* 推拿; *qigong* 气功 and *taichi* 推拿; and acupuncture, moxibustion and 5-element music therapy |

approach as RCTs, and have been described separately. Evidence from non-controlled studies is more difficult to evaluate, therefore the approach was taken to describe the characteristics of the study, details of the intervention and any adverse events. References to included studies are indicated by a letter followed by a number. Studies of CHM are indicated by a "H" e.g. H1; studies of acupuncture and related therapies indicated by an "A" e.g. A1; studies of other CM therapies indicated by an "O" e.g. O1; and studies of combinations of CM therapies indicated by a "C" e.g. C1 (see Table 4.1).

# Search Strategy

Evidence was searched in English- and Chinese-language databases and the methods followed the Cochrane Handbook of Systematic Reviews.[1] English-language databases included PubMed, Excerpta Medica Database (Embase), Cumulative Index of Nursing and Allied Health Literature (CINAHL), Cochrane Central Register of Controlled Trials (CENTRAL) which included the Cochrane Library, and Allied and Complementary Medicine Database (AMED). Chinese-language databases included China BioMedical Literature (CBM), China National Knowledge Infrastructure (CNKI), Chongqing VIP (CQVIP) and Wanfang. Databases were searched from inception to September 2016. No restrictions were applied. Search terms were mapped to controlled vocabulary (where applicable), in addition to being searched as keywords.

To conduct a comprehensive search of the literature, searches were run according to the study design (reviews, controlled trials, non-controlled studies). This was done for each of the three intervention types (CHM, acupuncture and related therapies, and other CM therapies) resulting in nine searches in each of the nine databases:

1. CHM — reviews;
2. CHM — controlled trials (randomised and non-randomised);
3. CHM — non-controlled studies;
4. Acupuncture and related therapies — reviews;
5. Acupuncture and related therapies — controlled trials (randomised and non-randomised);
6. Acupuncture and related therapies — non-controlled studies;
7. Other CM therapies — reviews;
8. Other CM therapies — controlled trials (randomised and non-randomised);
9. Other CM therapies — non-controlled studies.

Studies of combination CM therapies were identified through the above searches. In addition to electronic databases, reference lists of systematic reviews and included studies were searched for additional publications. Clinical trial registries were searched to identify clinical trials which were ongoing or completed, and where required, trial investigators were contacted to obtain data. The searched trial registries included the Australian New Zealand Clinical Trial Registry (ANZCTR), the Chinese Clinical Trial Registry (ChiCTR), the European Union Clinical Trials Register (EU-CTR), and the USA National Institutes of Health register (ClinicalTrials.gov). If required, trial investigators were contacted to obtain further information. Trial investigators were contacted by email or telephone, and were followed up after two weeks if no reply was received. Where no response was received after one month, any unknown information was marked as not available.

## Inclusion Criteria

- Participants: Adults diagnosed with major depression, also known as unipolar depression, diagnosed according to one of the following guidelines: Diagnostic and Statistical Manual of Mental Disorders (DSM),[2] Chinese Classification of Mental Disorders (CCMD),[3] or the International Classification of Disease (ICD).[4] Postpartum depression diagnosed by trained professional using the DSM, CCMD, or ICD. Aged 18 years to 65 years;
- Interventions: CHM, acupuncture and related therapies, or other CM therapies (Table 4.1). Integrative medicine such as CHM plus pharmacotherapy was also investigated;
- Comparators: Placebo, conventional therapies recommended in guidelines, including pharmacotherapy and psychotherapies;
- Outcome measures: Studies reported at least one of the pre-specified outcome measures (Table 4.2).

### Table 4.2. Pre-specified Outcomes

| Outcome Categories | Outcome Measures |
|---|---|
| Measurement of depression symptoms | • Hamilton Rating Scale for Depression (HRSD);<br>• Montgomery–Asberg Depression Rating Scale (MADRS);<br>• Beck Depression Inventory (BDI);<br>• Symptom Checklist-90;<br>• Depression, Anxiety and Stress Scale (DASS);<br>• Self-rating Depression Scale (SDS);<br>• Profile of Mood States (POMS);<br>• Edinburgh Postnatal Depression Scale (EPDS);<br>• Other depression scales including effective rate from defined guidelines e.g. 中医病证诊断疗效标准. |
| Relapse and remission of depression | 1. Number of participants who relapsed;<br>2. Number of participants who achieved remission. |
| Quality of life | 1. WHO Quality of Life-BREF (WHOQOL-BREF);<br>2. Short Form Health Survey (SF-36). |
| Functional capacity | Social adjustment scales |
| Suicidality | Number of participants with feelings of suicidality |
| Adverse events | Number and type of adverse events<br>• Treatment Emergent Symptom Scale (TESS);<br>• Rating Scale for Side Effects — Asberg (SERS). |

## Exclusion Criteria

- Bipolar depression or persistent depressive disorder (dysthymic disorder);
- Depressive symptoms or depression caused by other mental or physical disorders;
- Depression caused by another medical condition, such as post-stroke depression, or the effects of a substance;
- Excluded interventions included CHM formulated as intravenous injection. Also St. Johns Wort was excluded if it was not the entire plant but an extract used in the Western herbal context and not following CM principles of treatment;
- Integrative medicine studies that used different therapies in the intervention group, compared to the control group.

# Outcomes

Pre-specified outcomes included symptom scales of depression, number of participants who relapsed or achieved remission, quality of life, functional capacity (e.g. social adjustment scales), suicidality, and adverse events. Measurement of depression was not restricted and results from all depression instruments were included. Popular scales include the Hamilton Rating Scale for Depression (HRSD) and the Montgomery–Asberg Depression Rating Scale (MADRS). However, other self-rated and clinician-rated scales are available and were also included (Table 4.2).

## Hamilton Rating Scale for Depression

The HRSD is a clinician rated scale used to measure depression severity in adults. The original version contains 17 items (HRSD-17) and each item is scored on a 3- or 5-point scale. A total score is generated out of 54, where higher scores indicate more severe depression.[5] Other versions, including the HRSD-21, HRSD-24 and HRSD-29, have more items and capture additional clinical information. In this research, included studies used the HRSD-17, HRSD-24 or HRSD non-specified version. The HRSD is widely used in hospital and outpatient settings and is the most common instrument used in clinical trials of antidepressant medications. It was developed in the 1960s and is still useful and popular today. Alternatives have been developed over the years which have some advantages and disadvantages depending on the setting.

## Montgomery–Asberg Depression Rating Scale

The MADRS measures the severity of depression. It was designed as an adjunct to the HRSD as a more sensitive tool for measuring changes in depression after treatment.[6] Scores of the HRSD and the MADRS are highly correlated. The overall score ranges from 0–60 and higher scores indicate more severe depression. A score of zero to six indicates normal or absence of symptoms; seven to 19 indicates mildly depressed; 20 to 34 indicates moderately depressed; and more than 34 indicates severely depressed.

## Beck Depression Inventory

The BDI is widely used as a self-reported scale for depression severity. It differs from the HRSD and MADRS because it measures depression severity using self-report, rather than clinician-report. It consists of 21 items and higher scores indicate more severe depression.[7] There are three versions of the BDI, including the original first published in 1961, the BDI-1A published in 1978, and the BDI-II published in 1996. The most recent version, BDI-II, is used for individuals aged 13 years and above. A score of 0–13 is considered to be minimal depression; 14–19 is mild depression; 20–28 is moderate depression; and 29–63 is severe depression.[8]

## Zung Self-rating Depression Scale

The SDS is a self-rated 20-item scale that assesses affective, psychological, and somatic symptoms. The total score is then divided by a maximum possible score of 80. The SDS index score range from 0.25 to

1, higher index indicates more severe depression. A score of 20–44 is considered to be normal; 45–59 indicates mild depression; 60–69 indicates moderate depression; and 70 or more indicates severe depression.[9]

## Edinburgh Postnatal Depression Scale

The EPDS is a self-reported 10-item scale to screen for postnatal depression. The total possible score is 30 and a score of 10 or more suggests mild or major depression may be present and higher scores indicate more severe depression.[10]

## Treatment Emergent Symptom Scale

The Treatment Emergent Symptom Scale (TESS) is a review of all body systems and documents the presence, absence, and intensity of 28 symptoms. For each symptom, 3 judgments are required: 1) Intensity of the symptom; 2) Its relationship to the drug, and 3) The action undertaken as a consequence of its presence. Higher TESS scores indicate more severe adverse events.[11]

## Rating Scale for Side Effects — Asberg

The SERS is a 14-item scale to record the side effects of antidepressants. Each item is scored between 0–3, and higher total scores indicate more severe side effects.

## World Health Organisation Quality of Life Scale Brief Version

The WHOQOL-BREF is a quality of life assessment that includes physical, psychological, social relationships, and environmental domains. Higher scores indicate higher quality of life.[12]

There are many other scales used in clinical practice and research. A definitive list was not developed, rather all scales were analysed. Table 4.2 includes the most common scales.

## Risk of Bias Assessment

Risk of bias was assessed for RCTs using the Cochrane Collaboration's tool.[1] In clinical trials, bias can be categorised as selection bias, performance bias, detection bias, attrition bias, and reporting bias. Each domain is assessed to determine whether the bias is at "low", "high", or "unclear" risk. "Low" risk of bias indicates that bias is unlikely, "high" risk indicates plausible bias that seriously weakens confidence in the results and "unclear" bias indicates lack of information or uncertainty over potential bias, and raises some doubt about the results. Risk of bias assessment was verified by two people and disagreement was resolved by discussion or consultation with a third person.

Risk of bias is categorised using the following six domains:

- Sequence generation: The method used to generate the allocation sequence is given in sufficient detail to allow an assessment of whether it should produce comparable groups. "Low" risk of bias refers to a random number table or computer random generator. "High" risk of bias includes studies that describe a non-random sequence generation, such as odd or even date of birth or date of admission;
- Allocation concealment: The method used to conceal the allocation sequence is given in enough detail to determine whether intervention allocations could have been foreseen before, or during, enrolment. "Low" risk of bias includes central randomisation or sealed envelopes and "high" risk of bias includes open random sequence, etc;
- Blinding of participants and personnel: Measures used to describe if the study participants and personnel are blind to the intervention received. In addition, information relating to whether the blinding was effective is also assessed. Studies that ensure blinding of participants and personnel are at "low" risk of bias. If the study is not blind, or incompletely blind, it is at "high" risk of bias.
- Blinding of outcome assessors: Measures used to describe if the outcome assessors are blind to knowledge of which intervention a participant received. In addition, information relating to whether

the blinding was effective is also assessed. Studies that ensure blinding of outcome assessors are at "low" risk of bias. If the study is not blind, or incompletely blind, it is at "high" risk of bias.

- Incomplete outcome data: Completeness of outcome data for each main outcome, including dropouts, exclusions from the analysis with numbers missing in each group and reasons for dropout or exclusions. Studies with "low" risk of bias would include all outcome data, or if there is missing data, it is unlikely to relate to the true outcome or is balanced between groups. Studies at "high" risk of bias would have unexplained missing data.

- Selective reporting: The study protocol is available and the pre-specified outcomes are included in the report. Studies with a published protocol who include all pre-specified outcomes in their report would be at "low" risk of bias. Studies at "high" risk of bias would not include all pre-specified outcomes, or the outcome data may be reported incompletely.

## Statistical Analyses

Frequency of CM syndromes, CHM formulae, herbs and acupuncture points reported in the included studies are presented using descriptive statistics. The 10 most frequently reported CHM formulae and 20 most frequently reported herbs are presented. The top 10 acupuncture points used in two or more studies are presented, or as available. Where data was limited, reports of single CM syndromes or acupuncture points are provided as a guide for the reader.

Definitions of statistical tests and results are described in the glossary. Dichotomous data are reported as a risk ratio (RR) with 95% confidence intervals (CI), and continuous data are reported as mean difference (MD) or standardised mean difference (SMD) with 95% CI. For dichotomous data, when the RR is greater than one and the upper and lower values of the 95% CI are both greater than one, this indicates we can be 95% certain that there is a difference between the groups and that the true effect lies within these CIs. The same is true for values less than one. In such cases, we say there is a "significant difference" between the groups. For continuous data, when the MD is greater than zero and both the upper and lower values of the 95% CI are greater than zero, we say there is a "significant difference" between the groups. The same is true on the negative side of the scale.[1] For all analyses, RR or MD and 95% CI are reported, together with a formal test for heterogeneity using the $I^2$ statistic. An $I^2$ score greater than 50% was considered to indicate substantial heterogeneity.[1]

Sensitivity analyses were undertaken to explore potential sources of heterogeneity, based on "low" risk of bias for the risk of bias domain, sequence generation. Where possible and appropriate, planned subgroup analyses included duration of treatment, CM formula(e), comparator type and aetiology, including postpartum depression and menopausal depression. Available case analysis with a random effects model was used in all analyses to take into account the clinical heterogeneity likely to be encountered within and between included studies, and the variation in treatment effects between included studies.

## Assessment Using Grading of Recommendations Assessment, Development and Evaluation

The Grading of Recommendations Assessment, Development and Evaluation (GRADE) approach was used.[13] The GRADE approach summarises and rates the certainty of evidence in systematic reviews using a structured process for presenting evidence summaries. The results are presented in summary of findings tables. The results provide an important overview for depression outcomes.

A panel of experts was established to evaluate the evidence. The panel included the systematic review team, CM practitioners, integrative medicine experts, research methodologists, and conventional medicine physicians. The experts were asked to rate the clinical importance of key interventions from CHM, acupuncture therapies and other CM therapies, as well as comparators and outcomes. Results were collated and based on the rating scores and subsequent discussion, a consensus on the content for the summary of findings tables was achieved.

The certainty of evidence for each outcome was rated according to five factors outlined in the GRADE approach. The evidence may be rated based on:

- Limitations in study design (risk of bias);
- Inconsistency of results (unexplained heterogeneity);
- Indirectness of evidence (interventions, populations and outcomes important to the patients with the condition);
- Imprecision (uncertainty about the results);
- Publication bias (selective publication of studies).

These five factors are additive and a reduction in more than one factor will reduce the certainty of the evidence for that outcome. The GRADE approach also includes three domains that can be rated up, including a large magnitude of effect, dose-response gradient and effect of plausible residual confounding. However, these three domains relate to observational studies including cohort, case-control, before-after, time-series studies, and etc. GRADE summaries in this monograph only include RCTs, therefore these three domains for rating up were not assessed.

Treatment recommendations can also be assessed using the GRADE approach, but due to the diverse nature of CM practice, treatment recommendations were not included with the summary of findings. Therefore, the reader should interpret the evidence with reference to the local practice environment. It should also be noted that the GRADE approach requires judgments about the evidence and some subjective assessment. However, the experience of the panel members suggests the judgments are reliable and transparent representations of the certainty of evidence.

The GRADE levels of evidence are grouped into four categories:

1) "High" certainty evidence: We are very confident that the true effect lies close to that of the estimate of the effect;
2) "Moderate" certainty evidence: We are moderately confident in the effect estimate — The true effect is likely to be close to the estimate of the effect, but there is a possibility that it is substantially different;

3) "Low" certainty evidence: Our confidence in the effect estimate is limited — The true effect may be substantially different from the estimate of the effect;

4) "Very low" certainty evidence: We have very little confidence in the effect estimate — The true effect is likely to be substantially different from the estimate of effect.

## References

1. Higgins J and Green S. (eds.) (2011) Cochrane Handbook for Systematic Reviews of Interventions Version 5.1.0 (The Cochrane Collaboration). Retrieved from http://www.cochrane-handbook.org.

2. American Psychiatric Association. (2013) Diagnostic and Statistical Manual of Mental Disorders, 5th ed. American Psychiatric Publishing, Arlington, USA.

3. Chinese Society of Psychiatry. (2011) Chinese Classification of Mental Disorders (CCMD-3), 3rd ed. Shandong Science Technology Press, Jinan, People's Republic of China.

4. World Health Organization. (1992) International Statistical Classification of Diseases and Related Health Problems (ICD-10), 10th ed. World Health Organization, Geneva Switzerland.

5. Hamilton M. (1960) A rating scale for depression. *J Neurol Neurosurg Psychiatry* **23**(1): 56–62.

6. Montgomery SA and Asberg M. (1979) A new depression scale designed to be sensitive to change. *B J Psychiatry* **134**: 382–389.

7. Beck AT, Ward CH, Mendelson M, *et al.* (1961) An inventory for measuring depression. *Arch Gen Psychiatry* **4**: 561–571.

8. Beck AT, Steer RA, Ball R, and Ranieri W. (1996) Comparison of Beck Depression Inventories -IA and -II in psychiatric outpatients. *J Pers Assess* **67**(3): 588–597.

9. Zung WW. (1965) A self-rating depression scale. *Arch Gen Psychiatry* **12**: 63–70.

10. Cox JL, Holden JM, and Sagovsky R. (1987) Detection of postnatal depression. Development of the 10-item Edinburgh Postnatal Depression Scale. *Br J Psychiatry* **150**: 782–786.

11. National Institute of Mental Health. (1985) TESS (Treatment Emergent Symptom Scale-Write-in). *Psychopharmacol Bull* **21**: 1069–1072.

12. Harper H, Power M, and Group TW. (1998) Development of the World Health Organization WHOQOL-BREF quality of life assessment. *Psychol Med* **28**: 551–558.

13. Schunemann H, Brozek J, Guyatt G, and Oxman A. (eds.) (2013) GRADE handbook for grading quality of evidence and strength of recommendations (The GRADE Working Group). Retrieved from http://www.guidelinedevelopment.org/handbook/.

# 5

# Clinical Evidence for Chinese Herbal Medicine

## OVERVIEW

Chinese herbal medicine has been used and researched for its effects in improving depression and related symptoms. This chapter evaluates 121 clinical studies of Chinese herbal medicine for depression and includes 106 formulae and 145 herbs. The meta-analyses of randomised controlled trials indicate Chinese herbal medicine offers promising benefits, in terms of depressive and physical symptoms, in people with depression. In addition, Chinese herbal medicine appears to be safe and well tolerated by people with depression.

## Introduction

Chinese herbal medicine (CHM) for depression includes decoctions, granules, solutions, tablets, and capsules. Many different herb combinations and formulae have been used to treat depression and the most commonly evaluated in clinical trials are presented in this chapter.

## Previous Systematic Reviews

Previously, eight systematic reviews and meta-analyses have evaluated the efficacy of CHM, either alone, or in combination with conventional medicine for depression. In 2009, Zhao *et al.* reviewed all types of CHM for depression and included 18 randomised controlled trials (RCTs) (1,260 participants).[1] The results showed CHM was not superior in terms of reducing depression severity, compared to conventional medicine alone, or combined with other therapies or placebo.

In 2013, Butler *et al.* published a review of systematic reviews of CHM for depression including five published systematic reviews.[2] These systematic reviews focused on specific herbal formulae, including: *Xiao yao san* 逍遥散, modified *Xiao yao san* 逍遥散, and *Chai hu shu gan san* 柴胡疏肝散, as well as adjunctive use of Chinese herbs. A supplementary systematic review of studies published in English databases identified a further eight studies (756 participants). The authors of the review noted that, despite mentioning randomisation, most studies did not describe the details of randomisation. The authors also indicated the limitations of the studies in the methodology and reporting. Therefore, the efficacy of CHM for depression could not be confirmed.

In 2014, Yeung *et al.* reported the efficacy and safety of CHM for depression.[3] The systematic review included 296 studies (24,867 participants). A total of 345 CHM formulae were used in the studies. Most formulae were standardised and about one-third were individualised based on patient symptoms and CM syndromes. The most common formulae were: *Xiao yao san* 逍遥散, *Chai hu shu gan san* 柴胡疏肝散 and *Gan mai da zao tang* 甘麦大枣汤, and the frequently used herbs were *chai hu* 柴胡, *bai shao* 白芍 and *fu ling* 茯苓. The quality of all studies was assessed by modified Jadad scale and Cochrane's assessment tool. However, most studies had poor methodological quality. The meta-analysis showed that CHM was superior to placebo. Significant differences were not found between CHM (alone, or as a co-therapy) and antidepressants, in terms of the Hamilton Rating Scale for Depression (HRSD). As for safety, CHM had fewer adverse events (AEs) than antidepressants and there was no significant difference between placebo and CHM in the number of AEs. The use of combinations of CHM and antidepressants had fewer AEs compared with antidepressants alone. The authors indicated that, although the overall result was positive, it was premature to confirm the efficacy of CHM for depression because there were a small number of "high" quality studies.

Yeung *et al.* also reviewed the efficacy and safety of *Gan mai da zao tang* 甘麦大枣汤 alone, and as a co-therapy for depression and concurrent conditions, such as diabetes and post stroke depression in 2014.[4] Ten RCTs, including 968 participants, were included. The primary outcome measures were effective rate and self-rated or clinician-rated scales for depression severity. Results indicated that *Gan mai da zao tang* 甘麦大枣汤 combined with antidepressants could increase clinical efficacy and decrease the occurrence of AEs. As for safety, *Gan mai da zao tang* 甘麦大枣汤 had fewer AEs than antidepressants. However, the authors indicated that further high-quality studies with better methodology should be conducted because the number of *Gan mai da zao tang* 甘麦大枣汤 studies was small and the comparative effect size was very small.

Yeung *et al.* also published a systematic review of CHM for depression based on Chinese medicine (CM) syndromes.[5] This review was part of two of the previous systematic reviews above. A total of 61 studies, including 2,504 participants, were included. Syndromes were diverse, including 27 distinct groups for depression; the four most common were Liver *qi* depression, Liver depression and Spleen deficiency, and dual deficiency of the Heart and Spleen alongside Liver depression. Authors only analysed the four most common syndromes found in 42 studies. *Xiao yao san* 逍遥散 and *Chai hu shu gan san* 柴胡疏肝散 were commonly used for syndromes of Liver *qi* depression, Liver depression with Spleen deficiency, and Liver depression with *qi* stagnation. *Bai shao* 白芍 and *chai hu* 柴胡 were the most commonly used herbs. The results indicated that there was not sufficient evidence that certain formulae had greater effects for specific syndromes. Authors supposed the main reason was that there were only a limited number of studies on syndrome-based treatment for depression, of which methodological quality was "low".

In 2014, Jun *et al.* also evaluated the efficacy and safety of *Gan mai da zao tang* 甘麦大枣汤 for depression by conducting a systematic review and meta-analysis.[6] This review included a wide range of depression types including: major depression, melancholia, post-stroke depression, postpartum depression, involutional depression, and senile depression. Thirteen RCTs were included and pooled results showed *Gan mai da zao tang* 甘麦大枣汤 was not superior to antidepressants for any of the depression types, except post-stroke depression, although the evidence was at "high" risk of bias.

In 2014, Peng *et al.* reviewed *Wuling capsule* 乌灵胶囊 for post-stroke depression.[7] A total of 16 studies, including 1,378 participants, were included. The majority of studies were judged to have moderate methodological quality. Meta-analyses on HRSD, response rate, and AEs were conducted. The pooled results indicated *Wuling capsule* 乌灵胶囊, either alone or combined with pharmacotherapy, was effective. *Wuling capsule* 乌灵胶囊 integrated with antidepressants was superior to antidepressants alone, and reduced AEs. The authors suggested large sample-sized studies with rigorous design should be performed to further confirm the results.

In 2015, Ren *et al.* reviewed CHM for primary depression, post-stroke depression, and other secondary depression compared with fluoxetine.[8] A total of 26 studies, including 3,294 participants, were included. The pooled results showed CHM, for both primary and secondary depression, was as effective as 20 mg of fluoxetine per day, in terms of reducing HRSD scores. CHM had less AEs compared with fluoxetine. However, the authors indicated that the efficacy and safety of CHM for depression could not be confirmed because there was a limited number of "high" quality studies and bias was detected in the included studies.

## Identification of Clinical Studies

Database search identified 26,919 citations. After removing duplicates, excluding ineligible studies by reviewing the titles, abstracts and full text, a total of 121 clinical studies, including 10,095 participants, were finally included in the systematic review (Figure 5.1).

Records identified through other sources
(*n* = 0)

Records identified through English language database searching
(*n* = 24,567)

Records identified through Chinese language database searching
(*n* = 17,375)

Records after duplicates removed
(*n* = 26,919)

Records screened
(*n* = 26,919)

Records excluded (*n* = 24,701)

Full-text articles assessed for eligibility
(*n* = 2,218)

Full text articles excluded, with reasons (*n* = 2,097):

- Not a clinical study (*n* = 238)
- Not unipolar depression *n* = 188)
- Inappropriate diagnosis (*n* = 347)
- Inappropriate age range (*n* = 293)
- No outcomes of interest (*n* = 207)
- Inappropriate comparators (*n* = 59)
- Not CHM (*n* = 225)
- Inappropriate control (*n* = 440)
- Duplicate literature (*n* = 69)
- Full text unavailable (*n* = 9)
- Unsuitable data (*n* = 22)

Randomised controlled trials (*n* = 104)

Non-randomised controlled trials (*n* = 4)

Non-controlled studies
(*n* = 13)

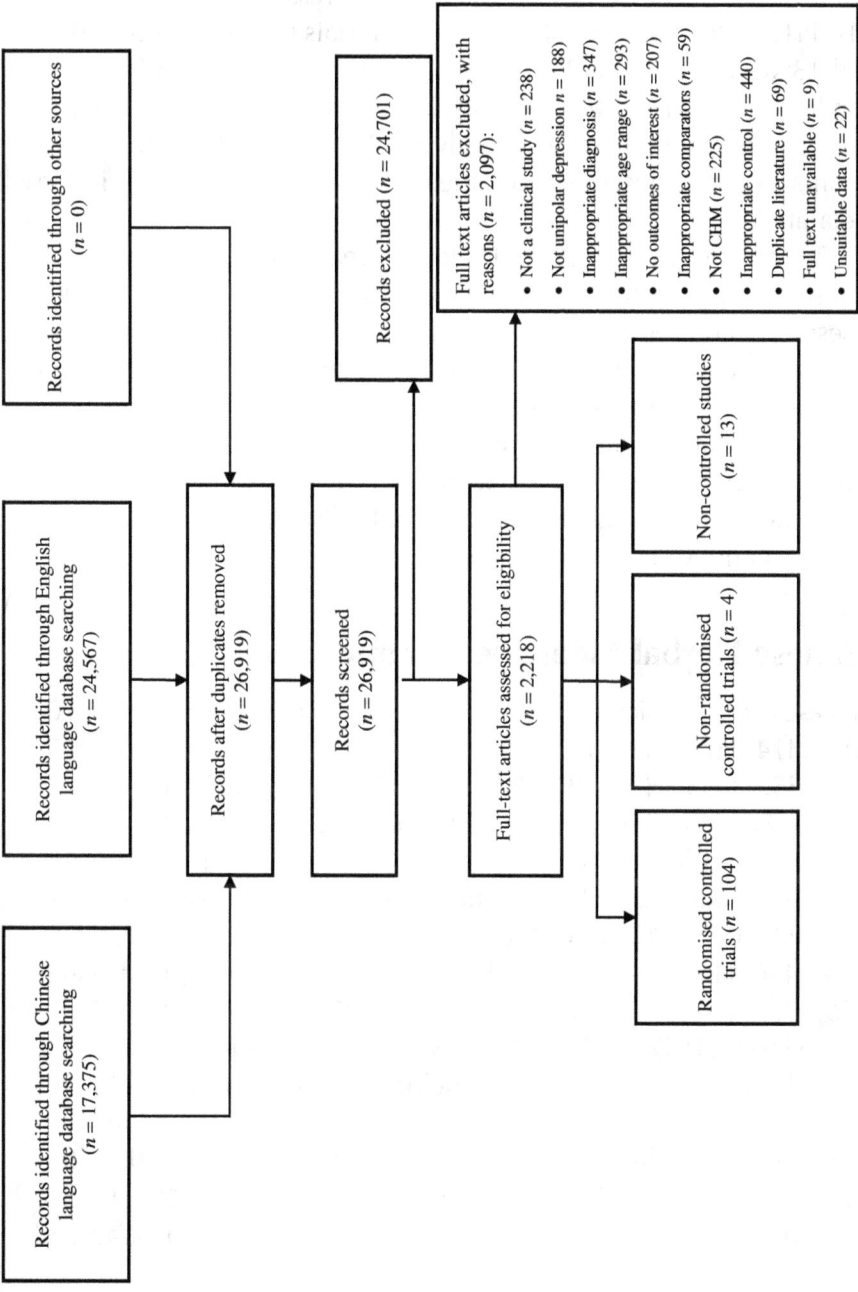

**Figure 5.1.** Flow Chart of Study Selection Process: Chinese Herbal Medicine

Among all clinical studies on CHM for depression, 104 were RCTs (H1–H104), four were controlled clinical trials (CCTs) (H105–H108) and 13 were non-controlled studies (H109–H121). All studies were conducted in China. Effects of CHM generated from RCTs and CCTs were synthesised using meta-analyses. Non-controlled studies are summarised and described, but their results are not included in the meta-analysis.

Participants ranged from 18 to 65 years of age. The average course of depression ranged from two weeks to 15 years. All studies assessed major depressive disorder alone and comorbid depression, such as post-stroke, were not included. In studies that described CM syndromes, the most common syndrome was Liver *qi* stagnation. Other common syndromes included Heart and Spleen deficiency, Liver *qi* stagnation with Spleen deficiency, *qi* stagnation transforming into heat, phlegm stagnation, melancholy disturbing the mind, and the Heart and Kidneys not interacting.

## Chinese Herbal Medicine Treatments

Chinese herbal medicine alone was assessed in 69 studies (H2, H6–H10, H12–H14, H21, H24, H27, H30–H34, H37, H39–H41, H45, H47, H49–H52, H55, H57–H60, H63, H64, H66, H67, H69, H70, H72, H75, H77, H82–H84, H86, H88, H90, H91, H93, H95–H101, H103–H106, H109–H121) and 52 studies combined CHM with conventional medicine including pharmacotherapy and psychotherapy (H1, H3–H5, H11, H15–H20, H22, H23, H25, H26, H28, H29, H35, H36, H38, H42–H44, H46, H48, H53, H54, H56, H61, H62, H65, H68, H71, H73, H74, H76, H78–H81, H85, H87, H89, H92, H94, H102, H107, H108). All CHM treatments were orally administrated. Oral preparation types included decoction, oral solution, capsules, granules, pills, and tablets. A total of 106 distinct formulae and 145 different herbs were investigated in the clinical studies. The most common formulae were: *Chai hu shu gan san* 柴胡疏肝散 (7 studies), *Dan zhi xiao yao san* 丹栀逍遥散 (4 studies), *Xiao yao san/wan* 逍遥散/丸 (4 studies), *Bu shen shu gan hua yu tan*g 补肾疏肝化瘀汤 (2 studies), *An shen ding zhi tang* 安神定志汤 (2 studies), and *Jia wei xiao yao capsule* 加味逍遥胶囊 (2 studies). The most frequent herbs were: *Chai hu* 柴胡 (88), *fu ling/fu shen* 茯苓/茯神 (76), *shao yao* 芍药 (69), *gan cao* 甘草 (68), and *yu jin* 郁金 (46). Controls included waiting list, placebo, pharmacotherapies, and psychotherapies.

## Randomised Controlled Trials of Chinese Herbal Medicine

One hundred and four RCTs (H1–H104) assessing CHM for depression were identified from the search. Fifty-eight used CHM alone (H2, H6–H10, H12–H14, H21, H24, H27, H30–H34, H37, H39–H41, H47, H49–H52, H55, H57–H60, H63, H64, H66, H67, H69, H70, H72, H75, H77, H82–H84, H86, H88, H90, H91, H93, H95–H101, H103, H104); 43 combined CHM with antidepressants (integrative medicine) (H3, H4, H11, H15–H17, H19, H20, H22, H23, H25, H26, H28, H29, H35, H36, H38, H42–H44, H46, H48, H53, H54, H56, H61, H62, H65, H68, H71, H73, H74, H76, H78–H81, H85, H87, H89, H92, H94, H102); two (H5, H18) combined CHM with antidepressants and psychotherapy (integrative medicine); and one combined CHM with psychotherapy (H1). Two RCTs (H103 and H104) included four arms with CHM alone, acupuncture alone, combined CHM with acupuncture, and antidepressants. Comparators included placebo, antidepressants, psychotherapy, and antidepressants with psychotherapy.

In total, 9,225 participants were included in the RCTs; age ranged from 18 to 65 years. Treatment duration ranged from one week to 12 weeks. Ninety-four distinct formulae (88 named and 6 unnamed) were assessed in the studies and the most common was *Xiao yao san (wan)* 逍遥散 used in four studies (Table 5.1). A total of 139 distinct herbs were used in the formulae and the most common was *chai hu* 柴胡 (Table 5.2).

Table 5.1.  **Frequently Reported Formulae in Randomised Controlled Trials**

| Most Common Formulae | No. of Studies | Ingredients |
|---|---|---|
| Xiao yao san (wan) 逍遥散 (丸) | 4 | Chai hu 柴胡, dang gui 当归, shao yao 芍药, fu ling 茯苓, bai zhu 白术, bo he 薄荷, jiang 姜, and gan cao 甘草 (H50, H74, H80, H104) |
| Chai hu shu gan san 柴胡疏肝散 | 3 | Chai hu 柴胡, shao yao 芍药, xiang fu 香附, zhi ke 枳壳, dang gui 当归, chen pi 陈皮, chuan xiong 川芎, and gan cao 甘草 (H46, H58, H90) |
| Dan zhi xiao yao san 丹栀逍遥散 | 3 | Chai hu 柴胡, dang gui 当归, shao yao 芍药, fu ling 茯苓, bai zhu 白术, mu dan pi 牡丹皮, zhi zi 栀子, and gan cao 甘草 (H34, H35, H51) |
| Bu shen shu gan hua yu tang 补肾疏肝化瘀汤 | 2 | Xian mao 仙茅, yin yang huo 淫羊藿, nv zhen zi 女贞子, mo han lian 墨旱莲, chai hu 柴胡, zhi ke 枳壳, chuan xiong 川芎, and di long 地龙 (H67, H84) |
| An shen ding zhi tang 安神定志汤 | 2 | 1. Chai hu 柴胡, bai zhu 白术, fu ling 茯苓, shao yao 芍药, yu jin 郁金, yuan zhi 远志, bai he 百合, shi chang pu 石菖蒲, he huan pi 合欢皮, and gan cao 甘草 (H23); 2. plus dang gui 当归 (H76) |
| Jia wei xiao yao capsule 加味逍遥胶囊 | 2 | Chai hu 柴胡, dang gui 当归, shao yao 芍药, bai zhu 白术, fu ling 茯苓, gan cao 甘草, mu dan pi 牡丹皮, zhi zi 栀子, and bo he 薄荷 (H7, H93) |

Ingredients are referenced to the original studies. The use of some herbs may be restricted in some countries. Readers are advised to comply with relevant regulations.

Table 5.2.  **Frequently Reported Herbs in Randomised Controlled Trials**

| Most Common Herbs | Scientific Name | Number of Studies |
|---|---|---|
| Chai hu 柴胡 | *Bupleurum chinense* DC var. *scorzonerifolium* Willd | 75 (chai hu 柴胡; 73, and cu chai hu 醋柴胡; 2) |
| Fu ling/fu shen 茯苓/茯神 | *Poria cocos* (Schw.) Wolf | 65 (fu ling 茯苓; 52, and fu shen 茯神; 13) |
| Shao yao 芍药 | *Paeonia lactiflora* Pall. | 58 (shao yao 芍药; 3, bai shao 白芍; 53, and chi shao 赤芍; 2) |
| Gan cao 甘草 | *Glycyrrhiza spp.* | 57 (gan cao 甘草; 36, zhi gan cao 炙甘草; 19, and sheng gan cao 生甘草; 2) |

**Table 5.2.**  (*Continued*)

| Most Common Herbs | Scientific Name | Number of Studies |
|---|---|---|
| Dang gui 当归 | *Angelica sinensis* (Oliv.) Diels | 45 (dang gui 当归; 44, and chao dang gui 炒当归; 1) |
| Yu jin 郁金 | *Curcuma spp.* | 39 |
| Bai zhu 白术 | *Atractylodes macrocephala* Koidz. | 38 (bai zhu 白术; 35, chao bai zhu 炒白术; 2, and jiao bai zhu 焦白术; 1) |
| Suan zao ren 酸枣仁 | *Ziziphus jujuba* Mill. var. spinosa (Bunge) Hu ex H. F. Chou | 33 (suan zao ren 酸枣仁; 23, and chao suan zao ren 炒酸枣仁; 10) |
| Xiang fu 香附 | *Cyperus rotundus* L. | 32 (xiang fu 香附; 30, cu xiang fu 醋香附; 1, and zhi xiang fu 制香附; 1) |
| Yuan zhi 远志 | *Polygala tenuifolia* Willd. | 29 |
| Chuan xiong 川芎 | *Ligusticum chuangxiong* Hort. | 26 |
| Shi chang pu 石菖蒲 | *Acorus tatarinowii* Schott | 26 |
| Chen pi 陈皮 | *Citrus reticulata* Blanco | 24 |
| Zhi ke 枳壳 | *Citrus aurantium* L. | 23 |
| Zhi zi 栀子 | *Gardenia jasminoides* Ellis | 23 (zhi zi 栀子; 20, zhi zhi zi 炙栀子; 1, chao zhi zi 炒栀子; 1, and jiao zhi zi 焦栀子; 1) |
| He huan hua/he huan pi 合欢花/合欢皮 | *Albizia julibrissin* Durazz. | 19 (he huan hua 合欢花; 4, and he huan pi 合欢皮; 15) |
| Ban xia 半夏 | *Pinellia ternata* (Thunb.) Breit. | 18 (ban xia 半夏; 13, qing ban xia 清半夏; 1, and fa ban xia 法半夏; 4) |
| Di huang 地黄 | *Rehmannia glutinosa* Libosch. | 15 (sheng di huang 生地黄; 10, and shu di huang 熟地黄; 5) |
| Dan shen 丹参 | *Salvia miltiorrhiza* Bge. | 14 |
| Dang shen 党参 | *Codonopsis pilosula* Nannf. var. modesta (Nannf.) L. T. Shen | 13 |
| Jiang 姜 | *Zingiber officinale* Rosc. | 12 (sheng jiang 生姜; 8, gan jiang 干姜; 1, and wei jiang 煨姜; 3) |
| Bo he 薄荷 | *Mentha haplocalyx* Briq. | 12 |
| Bai he 百合 | *Lilium lancifolium* Thunbspp. | 11 |

*Note*: The use of some herbs may be restricted in some countries. Readers are advised to comply with relevant regulations.

# Risk of Bias

All RCTs were described as "randomised". However, only 39 (37.5%) described an appropriate method of random sequence generation. Eight (7.7%) described the method of allocation concealment, while 96 (92.3%) were judged at "unclear" risk of bias because they did not describe the details of allocation concealment. Blinding of participants and personnel was reported in 18 studies (17.3%) which were judged to be at "low" risk of bias and 85 studies (81.7%) judged as "high" risk. The method of blinding of outcome assessors was judged as "low" risk of bias in 22 studies (21.2%). All outcome data were available for the majority of studies, and 102 (98.1%) were assessed as "low" risk of bias. Selective outcome reporting was judged at "unclear" risk in all the studies. A summary of the assessment of bias is presented in Table 5.3.

# Results of Meta-analyses

In the following sections, the meta-analyses results are presented according to the outcome measure. For each outcome, studies are grouped by type of comparison, for instance, CHM versus placebo; CHM versus antidepressants; CHM plus antidepressants versus antidepressants as integrative medicine; and CHM plus psychotherapy versus psychotherapy. Subgroup analysis included studies with "low" risk of

**Table 5.3. Risk of Bias of Randomised Controlled Trials**

| Risk of Bias Domain | Low Risk n (%) | Unclear Risk n (%) | High Risk n (%) |
|---|---|---|---|
| Sequence generation | 39 (37.5) | 62 (59.6) | 3 (2.9) |
| Allocation concealment | 8 (7.7) | 96 (92.3) | 0 (0.0) |
| Blinding of participants | 18 (17.3) | 1 (1.0) | 85 (81.7) |
| Blinding of personnel | 18 (17.3) | 1 (1.0) | 85 (81.7) |
| Blinding of outcome assessors | 22 (21.2) | 2 (1.9) | 80 (76.9) |
| Incomplete outcome data | 102 (98.1) | 2 (1.9) | 0 (0) |
| Selective outcome reporting | 0 (0) | 104 (100) | 0 (0) |

bias for sequence generation, treatment duration (≤6 weeks and >6 weeks), comparator drug class and comparator drugs. Studies that evaluated postpartum depression and menopausal depression were also subgrouped. In addition, subgroup analysis for studies that assessed different versions of the HRSD was performed. The pre-specified subgroup analyses were conducted to explore heterogeneity.

## Hamilton Rating Scale for Depression

Eighty-five of the 104 studies (including 7,702 participants) assessed severity of depression using the HRSD. Lower scores on the HRSD indicate greater improvement. Overall meta-analysis for HRSD was performed at the end of treatment based on different comparators.

### *Chinese Herbal Medicine vs. Placebo*

One RCT (H69) with 68 participants compared CHM to placebo. Treatment duration was six weeks. The result showed CHM was superior to placebo (mean difference (MD): −11.6 points [−15.83, −7.37]).

### *Chinese Herbal Medicine vs. Antidepressants*

Forty-seven RCTs (n = 4,632) compared CHM with antidepressants (H2, H6–H10, H21, H24, H27, H30, H31–H34, H37, H39–H41, H45, H47, H49, H50–H52, H55, H57–H60, H64, H66, H67, H70, H72, H75, H77, H82–H84, H86, H88, H90, H91, H93, H95–H97). Five classes of drugs were used as comparators, including selective serotonin reuptake inhibitors (SSRIs), serotonin and norepinephrine reuptake inhibitors (SNRIs), tricyclic antidepressants (TCAs), and tetracyclic. Specific drugs included: Fluoxetine, paroxetine, sertraline, dulxetine, venlafaxine, imipramine, and maprotiline. Treatment duration ranged from four to 12 weeks.

The overall result indicated an improvement in the CHM group, greater than in the antidepressant group (standardised mean difference (SMD)) −0.26 [−0.40, −0.12], $I^2$ = 80.4%) (Table 5.4).

**Table 5.4. Chinese Herbal Medicine vs. Antidepressants: Hamilton Rating Scale for Depression**

| Group | Subgroup | No. of Studies (Participants) | Effect Size (SMD [95% CI], I2%) | Included Studies |
|---|---|---|---|---|
| Antidepressants | All studies | 47 (4,632) | −0.26 [−0.40, −0.12]*, $I^2$ = 80.4% | H2, H6–H10, H21, H24, H27, H30, H31–H34, H37, H39–H41, H45, H47, H49, H50–H52, H55, H57–H60, H64, H66, H67, H70, H72, H75, H77, H82–H84, H86, H88, H90, H91, H93, H95–H97 |
| Antidepressants | Low ROB SG | 13 (1,244) | −0.04 [−0.29, 0.21], $I^2$ = 73.7% | H7, H10, H24, H27, H34, H37, H51, H60, H77, H83, H86, H93, H95 |
| Treatment duration | ≤6 weeks | 31 (2,976) | −0.24 [−0.38, −0.09]*, $I^2$ = 69.4% | H2, H6, H8, H10, H24, H30–H32, H34, H37, H39, H40, H45, H47, H49–H52, H55, H57–H60, H64, H75, H82, H83, H90, H96, H97 |
| | >6 weeks | 16 (1,656) | −0.30 [−0.62, 0.02], $I^2$ = 89.0% | H7, H9, H21, H27, H33, H41, H66, H67, H70, H72, H77, H84, H86, H88, H91, H93 |
| Drug class | SSRIs | 41 (4,121) | −0.28 [−0.44, −0.13]*, $I^2$ = 81.6% | H2, H6, H7, H9, H10, H21, H24, H27, H30, H32, H33, H37, H39–H41, H45, H47, H50–H52, H55, H58–H60, H66, H67, H70, H72, H75, H77, H82–H84, H86, H88, H90, H91, H93, H95–H97 |
| | SNRIs | 3 (332) | −0.17 [−0.64, 0.30], $I^2$ = 73.9% | H31, H57, H64 |
| | TCAs | 1 (47) | −0.63 [−1.22, −0.05]* | H8 |
| | Tetracyclics | 2 (132) | 0.28 [−0.07, 0.63], $I^2$ = 0.0% | H34, H49 |

| | | | | |
|---|---|---|---|---|
| Specific antidepressants | Fluoxetine | 31 (3,411) | −0.33 [−0.51, −0.14]*, I² = 83.9% | H6, H9, H10, H24, H27, H30, H32, H33, H37, H39–H41, H47, H50–H52, H55, H58–H60, H66, H67, H70, H72, H75, H77, H83, H90, H91, H95, H97 |
| | Paroxetine | 8 (518) | −0.12 [−0.45, 0.22], I² = 71.4% | H2, H21, H45, H82, H84, H86, H88, H96 |
| | Sertraline | 2 (192) | −0.20 [−0.81, 0.41], I² = 73.6% | H7, H93 |
| | Venlafaxine | 2 (132) | −0.29 [−1.13, 0.55], I² = 82.7% | H31, H64 |
| | Imipramine | 1 (47) | −0.63 [−1.22, −0.05]* | H8 |
| | Maprotiline | 2 (132) | 0.28 [−0.07, 0.63], I² = 0.0% | H34, H49 |
| | Duloxetine | 1 (200) | 0.01 [−0.27, 0.29] | H57 |
| Depression subtypes | Postpartum depression | 3 (285) | −0.71 [−1.41, −0.02]*, I² = 86.3% | H24, H32, H96 |
| | Menopausal depression | 5(380) | −0.28 [−0.90, −0.34]*, I² = 87.1% | H21, H30, H67, H77, H84 |
| HRSD | HRSD-17 | 18 (1,935) | MD: −0.48 [−1.13, 0.18], I² = 68.4% | H2, H9, H21, H37, H47, H49, H51, H55, H59, H64, H66, H72, H75, H77, H82, H83, H86, H97 |
| | HRSD-24 | 20 (1,790) | MD: −1.10 [−2.20, 0.00], I² = 84.2% | H6–H8, H10, H27, H30, H31, H33, H34, H41, H45, H50, H60, H70, H84, H88, H90, H91, H93, H95 |

* Statistically significant.

Abbreviations: HRSD, Hamilton Rating Scale for Depression; MD, Mean difference; ROB, risk of bias; SC, sequence generation; SNRIs, serotonin and norepinephrine reuptake inhibitors; SMD, standardised mean difference; SSRIs, selective serotonin reuptake inhibitors; TCAs, tricyclic antidepressants.

- Subgroup analysis by low risk of bias for sequence generation
  Subgroup analysis of 13 studies (n = 1,244) that were judged at "low" risk of bias for sequence generation was performed. It showed there was no statistical difference (SMD: −0.04 [−0.29, 0.21], $I^2$ = 73.7%]) (H7, H10, H24, H27, H34, H37, H51, H60, H77, H83, H86, H93, H95).

- Subgroup analysis by treatment duration
  Treatment duration for six weeks or less in 31 studies (n = 2,976) favored CHM, compared with antidepressants (SMD: −0.24 [−0.38, −0.09], $I^2$ = 69.4%) (H2, H6, H8, H10, H24, H30–H32, H34, H37, H39, H40, H45, H47, H49–H52, H55, H57–H60, H64, H75, H82, H83, H90, H96, H97). Sixteen RCTs, including 1,656 participants, with treatments durations longer than six weeks showed no difference between CHM and antidepressants (SMD: −0.30 [−0.62, 0.02], $I^2$ = 89.0%) (H7, H9, H21, H27, H33, H41, H66, H67, H70, H72, H77, H84, H86, H88, H91, H93). Heterogeneity remained high in the subgroups.

- Subgroup analysis by drug class
  Selective serotonin reuptake inhibitors were used as a comparator in 41 of the 47 RCTs, including 4,121 participants (H2, H6, H7, H9, H10, H21, H24, H27, H30, H32, H33, H37, H39–H41, H45, H47, H50–H52, H55, H58–H60, H66, H67, H70, H72, H75, H77, H82–H84, H86, H88, H90, H91, H93, H95–H97). The results indicated that the severity of depression was reduced in people receiving CHM, compared to SSRIs (SMD: −0.28 [−0.44, −0.13], $I^2$ = 81.6%); although heterogeneity remained high in the subgroup. One study (H8), with 47 participants, assessed CHM vs TCAs, indicating CHM was superior (SMD: −0.63 [−1.22, −0.05]). There was no difference between CHM and other comparator antidepressant drug classes, including SNRIs (H31, H57, H64) and Tetracyclics (H34, H49).

- Subgroup analysis by specific antidepressants
  Chinese herbal medicine reduced depression severity greater than fluxetine in 31 studies (n = 3,411) (SMD: −0.33 [−0.51, −0.14], $I^2$ = 83.9%) (H6,

H9, H10, H24, H27, H30, H32, H33, H37, H39–H41, H47, H50–H52, H55, H58–H60, H66, H67, H70, H72, H75, H77, H83, H90, H91, H95, H97). No statistical difference was seen when CHM was compared with other drugs, and heterogeneity remained "high" (H2, H7, H8, H21, H31, H34, H45, H49, H57, H64, H82, H84, H86, H88, H93, H96).

- Subgroup analysis for postpartum depression
  Three RCTs included 285 participants with postpartum depression. Treatment duration ranged from four to six weeks. All studies used SSRIs as comparators, including fluoxetin and paroxetine. The pooled results favoured CHM, although heterogeneity was substantial (SMD: −0.71 [−1.41, −0.02], $I^2$ = 86.3%) (H24, H32, H96).

- Subgroup analysis for menopausal depression
  Five RCTs included 380 menopausal women with depression. Treatment duration ranged from six to 12 weeks. All studies compared CHM with SSRIs, including fluoxetin and paroxetine. Menopausal depression was improved by CHM compared with antidepressants (SMD: −0.28 [−0.90, −0.34], $I^2$ = 87.1%) (H21, H30, H67, H77, H84).

- Subgroup analysis by HRSD version
  Eighteen studies (n = 1,935) used the HRSD-17 to compare CHM with antidepressants, including fluoxetine, paroxetine, venlafaxine, and maprotiline. Treatment duration ranged from four to 12 weeks. The results showed there was no statistical difference between groups (MD: −0.48 [−1.13, 0.18], $I^2$ = 68.4%) (H2, H9, H21, H37, H47, H49, H51, H55, H59, H64, H66, H72, H75, H77, H82, H83, H86, H97).

Twenty studies (n = 1,790) evaluated the severity of depression using the HRSD-24 version. Comparators included SSRIs, SNRIs, TCAs, or tetracyclic antidepressants. Treatment duration ranged from four to 12 weeks. The pooled results showed CHM was not superior to antidepressants, and heterogeneity was substantial (MD: −1.10 [−2.20, 0.00], $I^2$ = 84.2%) (H6–H8, H10, H27, H30, H31, H33, H34, H41, H45, H50, H60, H70, H84, H88, H90, H91, H93, H95).

The reason for the heterogeneity in the subgroup analysis was unclear.

### Chinese Herbal Medical plus Antidepressants vs. Antidepressants: Integrative Medicine

Thirty-six RCTs, including 2,942 participants, assessed the effects of CHM plus antidepressants vs antidepressants alone (studies used the same antidepressants in both groups) (H3, H11, H16, H17, H19, H23, H25, H26, H35, H36, H38, H42–H44, H46, H48, H53, H54, H56, H61, H62, H65, H68, H71, H73, H74, H76, H78–H81, H85, H87, H89, H92, H94). The antidepressants included SSRIs, SNRIs, noradrenergic and specific serotonergic antidepressants (NaSSAs), TCAs, or Tetracyclics. Treatment duration ranged from four to 12 weeks. Chinese herbal medicine plus antidepressants was superior to antidepressants alone (SMD: –0.95 [–1.22, –0.67], $I^2$ = 91.7%). Pre-specified subgroup analysis was performed to explore the heterogeneity (Table 5.5).

- Subgroup analysis for "low" risk of bias for sequence generation
  Fourteen studies with 1,155 participants were judged at "low" risk of bias for sequence generation. Subgroup analysis showed depression severity reduced in the integrative medicine group, compared to antidepressants. However, heterogenity was "high" (SMD: –0.95 [–1.26, –0.64], $I^2$ = 83.5%) (H16, H19, H42–H44, H48, H54, H56, H61, H71, H73, H78, H89, H94).

- Subgroup analysis by treatment duration
  Treatment duration for six weeks or fewer was assessed in 21 studies (n = 1,537) and 15 studies (n = 1,405) had a treatment duration of more than six weeks. Integrative medicine improved depression, compared to antidepressants alone (≤6 weeks: SMD: –0.83 [–1.16, –0.50], $I^2$ = 89.1%) (H3, H19, H25, H26, H35, H36, H38, H46, H53, H54, H56, H62, H68, H71, H74, H76, H78, H80, H85, H89, H92), and (>6 weeks: SMD: –1.10 [–1.57, –0.63], $I^2$ = 93.8%) (H11, H16, H17, H23, H42–H44, H48, H61, H65, H73, H79, H81, H87, H94).

- Subgroup analysis by drug class
  Chinese herbal medicine combined with SSRIs was superior to SSRIs alone in 26 studies (n = 2,173) (SMD: –0.89 [–1.24, –0.55], $I^2$ = 92.7%)

**Table 5.5. Chinese Herbal Medicine Plus Antidepressants vs. Antidepressants: Hamilton Rating Scale for Depression**

| Group | Subgroup | No. of Studies (Participants) | Effect Size (SMD [95% CI, I2%]) | Included Studies |
|---|---|---|---|---|
| Antidepressants | All studies | 36 (2,942) | $-0.95$ [$-1.22$, $-0.67$]*, $I^2 = 91.7\%$ | H3, H11, H16, H17, H19, H23, H25, H26, H35, H36, H38, H42–H44, H46, H48, H53, H54, H56, H61, H62, H65, H68, H71, H73, H74, H76, H79–H81, H85, H87, H89, H92, H94 |
| Antidepressants | Low ROB SG | 14 (1,155) | $-0.95$ [$-1.26$, $-0.64$]*, $I^2 = 83.5\%$ | H16, H19, H42–H44, H48, H54, H56, H61, H71, H73, H78, H89, H94 |
| Treatment duration | ≤6 weeks | 21 (1,537) | $-0.83$ [$-1.16$, $-0.50$]*, $I^2 = 89.1\%$ | H3, H19, H25, H26, H35, H36, H38, H46, H53, H54, H56, H62, H68, H71, H74, H76, H78, H80, H85, H89, H92 |
|  | >6 weeks | 15 (1,405) | $-1.10$ [$-1.57$, $-0.63$]*, $I^2 = 93.8\%$ | H11, H16, H17, H23, H42–H44, H48, H61, H65, H73, H79, H81, H87, H94 |
| Drug class | SSRIs | 26 (2,173) | $-0.89$ [$-1.24$, $-0.55$]*, $I^2 = 92.7\%$ | H11, H16, H17, H25, H26, H35, H38, H42–H44, H53, H61, H65, H68, H71, H73, H74, H76, H78–H81, H87, H89, H92, H94 |
|  | SNRIs | 4 (314) | $-0.89$ [$-1.52$, $-0.27$]*, $I^2 = 85.3\%$ | H3, H23, H46, H56 |
|  | TCAs | 2 (186) | $-1.50$ [$-3.56$, $-0.56$]*, $I^2 = 97.3\%$ | H54, H85 |
|  | Tetracyclics | 1 (74) | $-1.08$ [$-1.57$, $-0.59$]* | H19 |
|  | NaSSA | 3 (195) | $-1.04$ [$-1.76$, $-0.33$]*, $I^2 = 80.6\%$ | H36, H48, H62 |
| Specific antidepressants | Citalopram | 2 (160) | $-0.72$ [$-1.23$, $-0.21$]*, $I^2 = 60.3\%$ | H42, H94 |
|  | Escitalopram | 1 (68) | $-0.66$ [$-1.14$, $-0.17$]* | H11 |
|  | Fluoxetine | 10 (759) | $-0.90$ [$-1.68$, $-0.11$]*, $I^2 = 95.8\%$ | H17, H25, H26, H53, H68, H74, H78, H87, H89, H92 |

(Continued)

**Table 5.5.** *(Continued)*

| Group | Subgroup | No. of Studies (Participants) | Effect Size (SMD [95% CI], I2%) | Included Studies |
|---|---|---|---|---|
| | Paroxetine | 8 (814) | −0.92 [−1.51, −0.34]*, I² = 93.2% | H38, H44, H61, H65, H71, H73, H79, H80 |
| | Sertraline | 5 (372) | −0.99 [−1.43, −0.55]*, I² = 75.3% | H16, H35, H43, H76, H81 |
| | Venlafaxine | 2 (139) | −1.00 [−2.15, 0.160], I² = 90.3% | H3, H46 |
| | Maprotiline | 1 (74) | −1.08 [−1.57, −0.59]* | H19 |
| | Duloxetine | 2 (175) | −0.80 [−1.74, 0.14], I² = 87.9% | H23, H56 |
| | Mirtazapine | 3 (195) | −1.04 [−1.76, −0.33]*, I² = 80.6% | H36, H48, H62 |
| | Doxepin | 1 (104) | −2.55 [−3.08, −2.03]* | H54 |
| | Clomipramine | 1 (82) | −0.46 [−0.90, −0.02]* | H85 |
| Depression subgroups | Postpartum depression | 6 (511) | −0.93 [−1.58 −0.27]*, I² = 91.5% | H26, H43, H54, H62, H74, H89 |
| | Menopausal depression | 1 (72) | MD: −1.16 [−2.34, 0.02] | H78 |
| HRSD | HRSD-17 | 21 (1,683) | MD: −3.07 [−3.80, −2.35]*, I² = 74.3% | H3, H11, H19, H25, H26, H35, H36, H38, H44, H53, H54, H62, H65, H71, H73, H74, H80, H81, H85, H89, H94 |
| | HRSD-24 | 10 (847) | MD: −2.15 [−3.23, −1.06]*, I² = 86.6% | H23, H42, H43, H46, H48, H56, H78, H79, H87, H92 |

* Statistically significant.

Abbreviations: HRSD, Hamilton Rating Scale for Depression; NaSSA, noradrenergic and specific serotonergic antidepressants; MD, Mean difference; ROB, risk of bias; SG, sequence generation; SMD, standardised mean difference; SNRIs, serotonin and norepinephrine reuptake inhibitors; SSRIs, selective serotonin reuptake inhibitors; TCAs, tricyclic antidepressants.

(H11, H16, H17, H25, H26, H35, H38, H42–H44, H53, H61, H65, H68, H71, H73, H74, H76, H78–H81, H87, H89, H92, H94). Chinese herbal medicine plus SNRIs, in four studies with 314 participants (H3, H23, H46, H56), and CHM plus NaSSAs in three studies with 195 participants (H36, H48, H62), were also superior to antidepressants alone (SMD: –0.89 [–1.52, –0.27]; I$^2$ = 85.3%, and SMD: –1.04 [–1.76, –0.33], I$^2$ = 80.6%, respectively). There was difference between CHM plus TCAs and TCAs alone in two studies with 186 participants (SMD: –1.50 [–3.56, –0.56], I$^2$ = 97.3%) (H54, H85).

- Subgroup analysis by specific antidepressants
  Chinese herbal medicine plus sertraline, compared with sertraline alone, reduced depression severity in five studies with 372 participants (SMD: –0.99 [–1.43, –0.55], I$^2$ = 75.3%) (H16, H35, H43, H76, H81). Four studies used CHM plus venlafaxine (H3, H46) and duloxetine (H23, H56), but showed no difference between interventions and controls.

- Subgroup analysis for postpartum depression
  Six RCTs included 511 participants with postpartum depression. Treatment duration ranged from four to eight weeks. Comparators were TCAs, SSRIs, and NaSSAs. One study with 104 participants (H54) combined CHM placebo and doxepin as the comparator. The pooled results showed integrative medicine was superior to antidepressants (SMD : –0.93 [–1.58 –0.27], I$^2$ = 91.5%), although heterogeneity was "high" (H26, H43, H54, H62, H74, H89).

- Subgroup analysis for menopausal depression
  One RCT with 72 participants (H78) assessed menopausal depression and used fluoxetine as the control. Treatment duration was four weeks. Results showed there was no statistical difference between the two groups (MD: –1.16 [–2.34, 0.02]).

- Subgroup analysis by HRSD version
  Twenty-one RCTs (n = 1,683) used the HRSD-17 version. The results favoured CHM integrative medicine, compared with antidepressants alone (MD: –3.07 [–3.80, –2.35], I$^2$ =74.3%) (H3, H11,

H19, H25, H26, H35, H36, H38, H44, H53, H54, H62, H65, H71, H73, H74, H80, H81, H85, H89, H94).

A total of 10 RCTs (n = 847) used the HRSD-24 version. The pooled results showed an additional benefit of CHM plus antidepressants, compared to antidepressants alone (MD: –2.15 [–3.23, –1.06], $I^2$ = 86.6%) (H23, H42, H43, H46, H48, H56, H78, H79, H87, H92).

The reasons for the statistical heterogeneity were not identifiable in the meta-analyses.

### Chinese Herbal Medicine plus Antidepressants and Psychotherapy vs. Antidepressants plus Psychotherapy

One RCT (H18) recruited 60 participants and compared CHM, antidepressants and psychotherapy to antidepressants and psychotherapy. The integrative medicine group was superior to control (MD: –0.96 [–1.50, –0.43]).

## Zung Self-rating Depression Scale

The Zung Self-rating Depression Scale (SDS) assesses affective, psychological and somatic symptoms. Overall scores range from 20 to 80, and lower scores indicate less severe depression.

### Chinese Herbal Medicine vs. Antidepressants

The SDS was assessed in seven RCTs (n = 420). Treatment duration ranged from three to nine weeks. Five studies used SSRIs, including fluoxetine and paroxetine, as comparators and two used imipramine and maprotiline. One study (H51) compared CHM plus maprotiline placebo with maprotiline plus CHM placebo. In the pooled studies, CHMs were superior to antidepressants (MD: –2.01 [–3.00, –1.02], $I^2$ = 19.0%) (H8, H39, H51, H55, H66, H82, H91). Subgrouping by drug class revealed that CHM, compared to SSRIs, was superior to SSRIs alone in five studies (n = 307) (MD: –1.63 [–2.68, –0.57], $I^2$ = 10.0%) (H39, H55, H66, H82, H91). Furthermore, three studies (n = 144) compared CHM with fluoxetine. Results showed CHM was superior to fluoxetine (MD: −1.88 [−2.66, −1.10], $I^2$ = 0.0%) (H39, H55, H66).

## Chinese Herbal Medicine plus Antidepressants vs. Antidepressants

Two RCTs (n = 214) of CHM plus antidepressants, compared with antidepressants alone, reduced SDS scores (MD: −7.25 [−8.48, −6.02], $I^2$ = 0.0%) (H15, H17).

## Montgomery–Asberg Depression Scale

Montgomery–Asberg Depression Scale (MADRS) scores range from zero to 60. Lower scores indicate less severe depressive symptoms.

## Chinese Herbal Medicine vs. Antidepressants

One RCT enrolled 62 participants and assessed MADRS (H64). Treatment duration was six weeks and venlafaxine (extended release) was used as a control. At the end of treatment there was no significant difference between the groups (MD: 0.60 [−0.54, 1.74]).

## Chinese Herbal Medicine plus Antidepressants vs. Antidepressants

One RCT with 113 participants compared CHM plus venlafaxine with venlafaxine alone for eight weeks (H20). The integrative medicine group reduced depression more than the venlafaxine group (MD: −0.70 [−0.94,−0.46]).

## Edinburgh Postnatal Depression Scale

The Edinburgh Postnatal Depression Scale (EPDS) has 10 items that was used to identify females with postpartum depression. Lower scores indicate fewer depressive symptoms.

### Chinese Herbal Medicine vs. Placebo

One study included 60 participants and showed that CHM was superior to placebo (MD: –2.67 [–3.91, –1.43]) (H63).

### Chinese Herbal Medicine vs. Antidepressants

One study (n = 150) compared CHM to fluoxetine over 6 weeks. CHM was superior to fluoxetine (MD: –1.95 [–3.30, –0.60]; $I^2$ = 0.0%) (H32).

### Chinese Herbal Medicine plus Antidepressants vs. Antidepressants

One study, including 98 participants, compared CHM plus amitriptyline with amitriptyline alone. CHM plus amitriptyline was superior after six weeks treatment (MD: –3.37 [–5.29, –1.45]) (H29).

### Chinese Herbal Medicine plus Psychotherapy vs. Psychotherapy

One RCT (n = 49) compared CHM plus psychotherapy with psychotherapy alone. The results showed a significant benefit by adding psychotherapy to CHM over 12 weeks (MD: –2.00 [–3.16, –0.84]) (H1).

## Effective Rate

Effective rate is a method to assess clinical treatment effects. The definition of effective rate is not standardised. However, one common criteria is from the "Standards of diagnosis and effect for diseases and syndromes in Chinese medicine" (CM Standards).[9] It classifies treatment effect into one of three categories: 1) Cured — depression and accompanied symptoms are gone; 2) Improved — depression and accompanied symptoms improve; or 3) Ineffective — no change. Five RCTs assessed effective rate according to the CM Standards.

### Chinese Herbal Medicine vs. Antidepressants

Two studies (n = 174) reported that participants receiving CHM were 2.93 times more likely to achieve an improvement in depression compared to those receiving antidepressants (Risk Ratio (RR): 2.93 [1.55, 5.53], $I^2$ = 0.0%) (H12, H13).

### Chinese Herbal Medicine plus Antidepressants vs. Antidepressants

Two RCTs (n = 160) assessed CHM plus antidepressants, compared with antidepressants alone. One used escitalopram as the comparator over eight weeks and the other used mirtazapine and vitamin D over six weeks. The pooled results showed no difference between the groups (RR: 1.59 [0.70, 3.62], $I^2$ = 7.5%) (H11, H62).

### Chinese Herbal Medicine plus Psychotherapy vs. Psychotherapy

One RCT enrolled 49 participants and compared CHM plus psychotherapy, to psychotherapy alone. Treatment duration was 12 weeks. No statistical difference was seen between the two groups (RR: 2.24 [0.66, 7.68]) (H1).

## Assessment Using GRADE

An assessment of the certainty of the evidence from RCTs was made using Grading of Recommendations Assessment, Development and Evaluation (GRADE). Interventions, comparators and outcomes to be included were selected based on a consensus process, described in Chapter 4. Comparisons were: CHM vs antidepressants and CHM plus antidepressants vs antidepressants. Evidence for CHM vs antidepressants was "low" to "moderate" certainty (Table 5.6). The results showed that CHM may reduce clinician and self-rated depression severity. Evidence for CHM plus antidepressants vs antidepressants were "low" certainty (Table 5.7). The results showed that CHM may reduce clinician and self-rated depression severity.

**Table 5.6.  GRADE: Chinese Herbal Medicine vs. Antidepressants**

| Outcomes | No. of Participants (Studies) | Certainty of the Evidence (GRADE) | Anticipated Absolute Effects | |
|---|---|---|---|---|
| | | | Risk with Antidepressants | Risk Difference with CHM |
| **Hamilton Rating Scale for Depression**<br>Treatment duration: Mean 6.8 weeks | 4,632<br>(47 RCTs) | ⊕⊕○○<br>LOW[1,2] | | SMD: **0.26 SD lower**<br>(0.40 lower to 0.12 lower) |
| **Self-rating Depression Scale**<br>Scale from 20 to 80;<br>Treatment duration: Mean 5.7 weeks | 420<br>(7 RCTs) | ⊕⊕⊕○<br>MODERATE[1] | The mean Self-rating Depression Scale was **40.16** points | MD: **2.01 points lower**<br>(3 lower to 1.02 lower) |
| **Adverse events** | 2,323<br>(21 RCTs) | | The CHM groups had a total of 339 AEs. The most common were dry mouth (57 cases), constipation (32 cases), and loss of appetite (23 cases). The antidepressant groups reported 734 AEs. The most common were dry mouth (139 cases), constipation (75 cases), and tremor (36 cases). CHM significantly improved SERS scores (MD: −3.64 [−4.72, −2.56], I² = 9.9%) compared with antidepressants, indicating less side effects. | |

*The risk in the intervention group (and its 95% confidence interval) is based on the assumed risk in the comparison group and the relative effect of the intervention (and its 95% CI).

Abbreviations: AEs, Adverse events; CHM, Chinese herbal medicine; CI: confidence interval; GRADE, Grading of Recommendations Assessment, Development and Evaluation; MD, mean difference; RCTs: randomised contolled trials; SD, Standard deviations; SERS, side effect rating scales of Asberg; SMD, standardised mean difference.

*Notes:*

1. Unclear sequence generation and allocation concealment. Lack of blinding of participants and personnel;
2. Considerable statistical heterogeneity.

*Study References:*

Hamilton Rating Scale for Depression (HRSD): H2, H6–H10, H21, H24, H27, H30, H31–H34, H37, H39–H41, H45, H47, H49, H50–H52, H55, H57–H60, H64, H66, H67, H70, H72, H75, H77, H82–H84, H86, H88, H90, H91, H93, H95–H97;
Self-rating Depression Scale (SDS): H8, H39, H51, H55, H66, H82, H91;

| Outcomes | No. of Participants (Studies) | Certainty of the Evidence (GRADE) | Anticipated Absolute Effects | |
|---|---|---|---|---|
| | | | Risk with Antidepressants | Risk Difference with CHM Plus Antidepressants |
| **Hamilton Rating Scale for Depression** Treatment duration: Mean 6.5 weeks | 2,942 (36 RCTs) | ⊕⊕◯◯ LOW[1,2] | | SMD: **0.95 SD lower** (1.22 lower to 0.67 lower) |
| **Self-rating Depression Scale** Scale from 20 to 80; Treatment duration: Mean 9 weeks | 214 (2 RCTs) | ⊕⊕◯◯ LOW[1,3] | The mean Self-rating Depression Scale was **51.65 points** | MD: **7.25 points lower** (8.48 lower to 6.02 lower) |
| **Adverse events** | 1,694 (21 RCTs) | | Integrative CHM group had a total of 257 AEs, the most common were constipation (32 cases), dry mouth (29 cases), and nausea and vomiting (28 cases). The antidepressant groups reported 409 AEs, the most common were constipation (58 cases), dry mouth (45 cases), and nausea and vomiting (36 cases). Integrative CHM significantly improved TESS scores (MD: −2.50 [−3.59, −1.41], I² = 98.3%) compared with antidepressants, indicating less AEs. | |

*The risk in the intervention group (and its 95% confidence interval) is based on the assumed risk in the comparison group and the relative effect of the intervention (and its 95% CI).

Abbreviations: AEs, Adverse events; CHM, Chinese herbal medicine; CI, confidence interval; MD, mean difference; RCTs, randomised controlled trials; SD, Standard deviations; SMD: standardised mean difference; TESS, Treatment Emergent Symptom Scale.

*Notes:*

1. Unclear sequence generation and allocation concealment. Lack of blinding of participants and personnel;
2. Considerable statistical heterogeneity;
3. Small sample size.

*Study References:*

Hamilton Rating Scale for Depression (HRSD): H3, H11, H16, H17, H19, H23, H25, H26, H35, H36, H38, H42–H44, H46, H48, H53, H54, H56, H61, H62, H65, H68, H71, H73, H74, H76, H79–H81, H85, H87, H89, H92, H94;
Self-rating Depression Scale (SDS): H15, H17;
Adverse events: H4, H16, H17, H19, H22, H23, H28, H29, H38, H42–H44, H46, H56, H61, H68, H73, H78, H80, H81, H102.

# Randomised Controlled Trial Evidence for Individual Formulae

Eighty-eight named formulae and 6 unnamed formulae were reported in 104 RCTs. Evidence for the top 10 individual formulae used in two or more studies are separately analysed.

## Xiao yao san/wan 逍遥散/丸

*Xiao yao san/wan* was evaluated in four studies (H50, H74, H80, H103). Data from three studies (H50, H74, H80) could be pooled in a meta-analysis for HRSD. Two studies (H74, H80) assessed AEs using the Treatment Emergent Symptom Scale (TESS) and two studies (H80, H103) calculated each comparator's AEs.

## Hamilton Rating Scale for Depression

*Xiao yao san* reduced depression severity but there was no significance, compared to fluoxetine, in one study with 48 participants (MD: −0.95 [−2.47, 0.57]) (H50). Two studies (n = 108) combined *Xiao yao wan* with antidepressants and it was superior to antidepressants alone (MD: −1.23 [−2.81, −0.35], I² = 0.0%) (H74, H80).

## Treatment Emergent Symptom Scale

*Xiao yao wan* was superior to antidepressants in terms of TESS in two studies (n = 108) (MD: −0.45 [−0.70, −0.19], I² = 0.0%) (H74, H80).

## Adverse Events

One study (n = 62) investigated *Xiao yao wan* combined with paroxetine, compared to paroxetine alone, and reported AEs (H80). The integrative medicine group had a total of 10 AEs, including nausea and vomiting (3), dizziness and headache (2), dry month (1), constipation (1), hypersomnia (1), blurred vision (1), and tremor (1). The antidepressant group reported 30 AEs including blurred vision

(12), nausea and vomiting (6), dry mouth (3), dizziness and headache (3), constipation (2), hypersomnia (2), and tremor (2). One three-arm study (n = 87) evaluated *Xiao yao san* compared with placebo reported bloating (1) as an AE in the CHM group.

## Chai hu shu gan san 柴胡疏肝散

*Chai hu shu gan san* was evaluated in three studies (H46, H58, H89).

## Hamilton Rating Scale for Depression

*Chai hu shu gan san* was more effective than fluoxetine in one study (n = 60) (MD: –2.80 [–4.35, –1.25]) (H58). Two studies (n = 150) also showed *Chai hu shu gan san* combined with antidepressants (venlafaxine, fluoxetine) was superior to antidepressants alone (MD: –0.39 [–0.72, –0.07], $I^2$ = 0.0%) (H46, H89).

## Adverse Events

One study (n = 63) compared *Chai hu shu gan san* plus venlafaxine, to venlafaxine alone (H46). The integrative group reported 24 AEs including sweating (6), constipation (5), hypertension (3), headache (3), nausea and vomiting (2), insomnia (2), hypersomnia (1), dry mouth (1), and blurred vision (1). The venlafaxine group had a total of 72 AEs including constipation (16), sweating (15), headache (9), insomnia (6), hypersomnia (6), hypertension (6), dry month (4), nausea and vomiting (4), blurred vision (3), and tremor (3).

## Dan zhi xiao yao san 丹栀逍遥散

*Dan zhi xiao yao san* was evaluated in three studies (H34, H35, H51).

## Hamilton Rating Scale for Depression

In terms of reducing depression severity *Dan zhi xiao yao san* was not superior to maprotiline in two studies with 132 participants (SMD: 0.28

[–0.07, –0.63], I² = 0.0%) (H34, H51). However, the integrative use of *Dan zhi xiao yao san* and sertraline was superior to sertraline alone in one study with 80 participants (MD: –2.7 [–3.41, –1.89]) (H35).

## Self-rating Depression Scale

Self-rating Depression Scale was measured in one study (n = 66) (H51). *Dan zhi xiao yao san* was not superior to maprotiline (MD: –1.19 [–10.84, 8.46]).

## Side Effect Rating Scales of Asberg

Only one study (n = 66) evaluated the safety of *Dan zhi xiao yao san* using the side-effect rating scales of Asberg (SERS) (H51). *Dan zhi xiao yao san* had less side effects compared to maprotiline (MD: –2.72 [–4.75, –0.69]).

## An shen ding zhi tang 安神定志汤

Two studies evaluated *An shen ding zhi tang* (H23, H76).

## Hamilton Rating Scale for Depression

Two studies (n = 190) assessed *An shen ding zhi tang* combined with antidepressants (duloxetine and sertraline) (H23, H76). Integrative medicine improved depression severity, compared to antidepressants alone (SMD: –0.36 [–0.64, –0.07], I² = 0.0%).

## Treatment Emergent Symptom Scale

One study (n = 80) evaluated safety by using the TESS (H76). *An shen ding zhi tang* combined with sertraline improved TESS scores more than sertraline alone (MD: –0.60 [–0.82, –0.38]).

## Adverse Events

One study (n = 110) reported AEs (H23). The *An shen ding zhi tang*, combined with duloxetine group, reported 17 AEs including hypertension (3), headache (3), nausea (3), dry mouth (2), loss of appetite (2), fatigue (2), insomnia (1), and constipation (1). The duloxetine group had a total of 19 AEs including insomnia (6), dry mouth (5), fatigue (3), constipation (2), nausea (2), and loss of appetite (1).

## Bu shen shu gan hua yu tang 补肾疏肝化瘀汤

*Bu shen shu gan hua yu tang* was evaluated in two studies (n=228) (H67, H84). *Bu shen shu gan hua yu tang* did not show improvement in HRSD scores when compared to fluoxetine or paroxetine (SMD: –0.55 [–1.64, 0.53], I² = 92.3%). The studies did not report on AEs.

## Jia wei xiao yao capsules 加味逍遥胶囊

*Jia wei xiao yao capsules* were evaluated in two studies (n = 192) (H7, H93).

## Hamilton Rating Scale for Depression

*Jia wei xiao yao capsules* were not superior to sertraline (SMD: –0.92 [–3.79, 1.95], I² = 71.7%) (H7, H93).

## Adverse Events

One study (n = 65) reported AEs (H7). The *Jia wei xiao yao* capsule group had one report of dry mouth and headache, while the sertraline group reported two AEs including dry mouth, nausea and dry eyes (2).

## Frequently Reported Used Herbs in Meta-analyses Showing Favourable Effect

The most frequently used herbs in meta-analyses showing favourable effect were calculated according to outcome category and comparator type. Table 5.8 includes the list of herbs.

**Table 5.8.** Frequently Reported Herbs in Meta-analyses Showing Favourable Effect

| Herb | Scientific Name | Number of Studies |
| --- | --- | --- |
| **Chinese Herbal Medicine vs. Antidepressants: Depression severity\*, 3 meta-analyses, 47 RCTs (Table 5.4)** | | |
| Chai hu 柴胡 | *Bupleurum chinense* DC | 32 |
| Fu ling/fu shen 茯苓/茯神 | *Poria cocos* (Schw.) Wolf | 25 (fu ling 23, fu shen 2) |
| Shao yao 芍药 | *Paeonia lactiflora* Pall. | 23 |
| Gan cao 甘草 | *Glycyrrhiza spp.* | 22 |
| Yu jin 郁金 | *Curcuma spp.* | 16 |
| Dang gui 当归 | *Angelica sinensis* (Oliv.) Diels | 15 |
| Yuan zhi 远志 | *Polygala tenuifolia* Willd. | 14 |
| Bai zhu 白术 | *Atractylodes macrocephala* Koidz. | 13 |
| Shi chang pu 石菖蒲 | *Acorus tatarinowii* Schott | 13 |
| Suan zao ren 酸枣仁 | *Ziziphus jujuba* Mill. var. *spinosa* (Bunge) Hu ex H. F. Chou | 13 |
| Zhi zi 栀子 | *Gardenia jasminoides* Ellis | 12 |
| Chuan xiong 川芎 | *Ligusticum chuangxiong* Hort. | 10 |
| **Chinese Herbal Medicine plus Antidepressants vs. Antidepressants: Depression severity\*, 4 meta-analyses, 39 RCTs (Table 5.5)** | | |
| Chai hu 柴胡 | *Bupleurum chinense* DC | 32 |
| Shao yao 芍药 | *Paeonia lactiflora* Pall. | 25 |
| Gan cao 甘草 | *Glycyrrhiza spp.* | 24 |
| Fu ling/fu shen 茯苓/茯神 | *Poria cocos* (Schw.) Wolf | 24 (fu ling 18, fu shen 6) |
| Dang gui 当归 | *Angelica sinensis* (Oliv.) Diels | 20 |
| Bai zhu 白术 | *Atractylodes macrocephala* Koidz. | 18 |
| Xiang fu 香附 | *Cyperus rotundus* L. | 18 |
| Yu jin 郁金 | *Curcuma spp.* | 17 |
| Suan zao ren 酸枣仁 | *Ziziphus jujuba* Mill. var. *spinosa* (Bunge) Hu ex H. F. Chou | 15 |
| He huan hua/he huan pi 合欢花/合欢皮 | *Albizia julibrissin* Durazz. | 12 |
| Chuan xiong 川芎 | *Ligusticum chuangxiong* Hort. | 12 |

Table 5.8. (*Continued*)

| Herb | Scientific Name | Number of Studies |
|------|-----------------|-------------------|
| Chen pi 陈皮 | *Citrus reticulata* Blanco | 12 |
| Zhi ke 枳壳 | *Citrus aurantium* L. | 11 |
| Shi chang pu 石菖蒲 | *Acorus tatarinowii* Schott | 10 |
| Yuan zhi 远志 | *Polygala tenuifolia* Willd. | 10 |

*Depression severity measured on the Edinburgh Postnatal Depression Scale (EPDS), Hamilton Rating Scale for Depression (HRSD), Montgomery–Asberg Depression Rating Scale (MADRS), or on Zung's Self-rating Depression Scale (SDS).

# Safety of Chinese Herbal Medicine in Randomised Controlled Trials

## Treatment Emergent Symptom Scale

For outcome measurements of safety, there were 10 RCTs that used the TESS, which was developed for assessing the presence and intensity of side effects. Lower scores of TESS indicate fewer side effects.

Ten pooled RCTs (n = 716) showed that integrative medicine was superior in reducing side effects compared with antidepressants alone (MD: –2.50 [–3.59, –1.41], $I^2$ = 98.3%) (H16, H20, H48, H54, H71, H74, H76, H80, H81, H92).

## Side Effect Rating Scales of Asberg

The SERS is a 15-item safety assessment covering somatic symptoms, headache, and dizziness. Lower SERS scores indicate decreased severity of side effects.

Two RCTs (n = 113) comparing CHM with antidepressants assessed SERS. There was lower severity of side effects in the CHM group, compared to antidepressants (MD: –3.64 [–4.72, –2.56], $I^2$ = 9.9%) (H8, H51).

## Adverse Events

Out of the 104 studies, 48 mentioned AEs. Of these, 43 studies provided specific details about the AEs (Table 5.9).

**Table 5.9.  Adverse Events**

| Intervention Group Adverse Events | Control Group Adverse Events |
|---|---|
| **Chinese Herbal Medicine vs. Placebo (4 studies)** | |
| Total Adverse Events = 20<br>Increased appetite (5), anxiety (3), headache (3), loss of appetite (2), nausea (2), hypomania (2), bloating (1), dry mouth (1), sedation (1) | Total Adverse Events = 12<br>Anxiety (1), decreased appetite (2), increased appetite (1), sedation (2), nausea (2), headache (2), hypomania (1), constipation (1) |
| **Chinese Herbal Medicine vs. Antidepressants (21 studies)** | |
| Total Adverse Events = 339<br>Dry mouth (57), constipation (32), loss of appetite (23), headache (20), nausea (17), tachycardia (15), blurred vision (14), tremor (10), increased appetite (9), anxiety (8), restlessness (5), sweating (5), dizziness (4), hypersomnia (4), tiredness (4), heart pounding (3), insomnia (3), nasal congestion (3), nausea and vomiting (3), sexual dysfunction (3), urinary retention (3), anxiety and nervousness (2), hypomania (2), abdominal pain (1), abnormal liver function (1), diarrhea (1), dry mouth and headache (1), low blood pressure (1), unspecified/others (85) | Total Adverse Events = 734<br>Dry mouth (139), constipation (75), tremor (36), loss of appetite (35), tachycardia (27), blurred vision (24), nausea (20), dizziness (18), increased appetite (16), urinary retention (13), headache (12), tiredness (12), low blood pressure (11), nausea and loss of appetite (7), sweating (11), insomnia (10), dizziness and headache (7), hypersomnia (7), sexual dysfunction (7), abnormal urine (6), anxiety (6), indigestion (6), sleep disorder (6), headache, nausea and vomiting (5), loss of appetite, dizziness, headache, abnormal sleep and tiredness (4), palpitation (4), anxiety and insomnia (3), disturbances of consciousness (3), excessive excitement or agitation (3), nausea and vomiting (3), nausea, vomiting, indigestion, diarrhea, and dysphasia (3), dry mouth, nausea and dry eyes (2), heart pounding (2), restlessness (2), abnormal mental state, sexual dysfunction, abnormal vision and dyspnoea (1), anxiety and nervousness (1), diarrhea (1), hyper-salivation (1), hypomania (1), urticaria (1), unspecified/others (183) |

**Table 5.9.** (*Continued*)

| Intervention Group Adverse Events | Control Group Adverse Events |
|---|---|
| **Chinese Herbal Medicine plus Antidepressants vs. Antidepressants (21 studies)** | |
| Total Adverse Events = 257<br>Constipation (32), dry mouth (29), nausea and vomiting (28), nausea (27), diarrhea (20), blurred vision (17), dizziness (15), hypersomnia (13), sweating (13), headache (10), insomnia (10), excessive stillness (7), loss of appetite (6), tremor (6), nausea and loss of appetite (3), tiredness (3), weight gain (3), hypertension (3), dizziness and headache (2), dizziness and palpitation (1), tachycardia (1), raised blood pressure (1), unspecified/others (7) | Total Adverse Events = 409<br>Constipation (58), dry mouth (45), nausea and vomiting (36), nausea (32), sweating (26), insomnia (25), hypersomnia (24), blurred vision (21), dizziness (16), diarrhea (14), headache (14), loss of appetite (13), tremor (13), excessive stillness (7), tiredness (6), hypertension (6), rash (4), nausea and loss of appetite (4), sexual dysfunction (4), weight gain (4), dizziness and headache (3), dizziness and palpitation (3), sleep disorder (3), nausea and dry mouth (2), vomiting (2), tachycardia (2), anxiety (1), palpitation (1), raised blood pressure (1), unspecified/others (19) |
| **Chinese Herbal Medicine plus Antidepressants and Psychotherapy vs. Antidepressants and Psychotherapy (2 studies)** | |
| Total Adverse Events = 10<br>Dizziness (1), indigestion (2), unspecified/others (7) | Total Adverse Events = 33<br>Dizziness (5), insomnia (3), indigestion (4), unspecified/others (21) |

## *Chinese Herbal Medicine vs. Placebo*

In four RCTs of CHM vs placebo, the total number of AEs reported in the CHM group was 20, and in the placebo group was 12. The most common AE in the CHM group was increased appetite (5 cases) followed by anxiety and headache (3 cases each) (H63, H100, H103, H104).

## *Chinese Herbal Medicine vs. Antidepressants*

In 21 studies comparing CHM with antidepressants, 339 AEs were reported in people who were allocated to receive CHM, and 734 AEs were reported in people who used antidepressants (H6, H7, H14, H24,

H27, H30, H32, H33, H41, H47, H49, H57, H60, H70, H77, H88, H90, H96, H98, H99, H101). Events included dry mouth, constipation and loss of appetite. One RCT (H77) reported on the number of AEs in each group but details of AEs were not specified. Another RCT (H41) reported the nature of the events but not the number of AEs in the antidepressant group. In the other 19 studies (H6, H7, H14, H24, H27, H30, H32, H33, H47, H49, H57, H60, H70, H88, H90, H96, H98, H99, H101), five reported no AEs and 14 reported information on 267 AEs in the CHM group. Dry mouth was the most commonly reported AEs (57 cases) followed by constipation (32 cases), loss of appetite (23 cases), and headache (20 cases). Other AEs included nausea, tachycardia, and blurred vision. In the antidepressant groups, 558 AEs were reported with detailed information, and common events included dry mouth (139 cases), constipation (75 cases), and tremor (36 cases).

## Chinese Herbal Medicine plus Antidepressants vs. Antidepressants

Twenty-one RCTs mentioned AEs when CHM plus antidepressants was compared with antidepressants alone (H4, H16, H17, H19, H22, H23, H28, H29, H38, H42–H44, H46, H56, H61, H68, H73, H78, H80, H81, H102). A total of 257 AEs were reported in the integrative medicine groups, while 409 AEs were reported in the antidepressant groups. Nineteen studies (H4, H16, H17, H19, H22, H23, H29, H38, H42–H44, H46, H56, H61, H68, H73, H80, H81, H102) provided AE information. Constipation was the most common AE in both the CHM and control groups (32 and 58 cases, respectively). Other AEs included nausea and vomiting (28 and 36 cases, respectively) and dry mouth (29 and 45 cases, respectively).

## Chinese Herbal Medicine plus Antidepressants and Psychotherapy vs. Antidepressants and Psychotherapy

Two studies (H5, H18) compared CHM plus antidepressants and psychotherapy to antidepressants and psychotherapy alone. Reported

AEs included indigestion (2 cases) and dizziness (1 case) in the integrative medicine group, and dizziness (5 cases), indigestion (4 cases), and insomnia (3 cases) in the control group.

# Controlled Clinical Trials of Chinese Herbal Medicine

Four controlled clinical trials investigated the effect of CHM in 225 participants (H105–H108). Two studies (H105, H106) evaluated CHM versus antidepressants and two studies (H107, H108) evaluated CHM and antidepressants vs antidepressants alone.

Treatment duration ranged from four to eight weeks. Three different Chinese herbal formulae and one single herb (*bai guo* 白果 *Ginkgo Biloba*) were used in the studies. All formulae were orally administrated. Twenty herbs were used in the formulae and the most common included *chai hu* 柴胡 and *gan cao* 甘草. The controls included fluoxetine in two studies (H105, H107), mirtazapine in one study (H106), and trimipramine in the other studies (H108).

## Hamilton Rating Scale for Depression

Four studies measured the HRSD. Two studies (n = 111) evaluated the effect of CHM compared with antidepressants, and CHM was not superior to antidepressants (MD: 0.04 [–2.51, 2.59], $I^2$ = 0.0%) (H105, H106).Two studies (n = 114) evaluated integrative CHM and antidepressants, compared to antidepressants alone (H107, H108). The integrative medicine group did not reduce depression severity compared to antidepressants (SMD: 0.10 [–1.85, 2.05], $I^2$ = 91.4%).

## Zung Self-rating Depression Scale

One study, with 16 participants, assessed symptoms of depression on the SDS (H108). Integrative CHM was not more effective at reducing depression than antidepressants alone (MD:10.12 [–4.66, 24.90]).

## Safety of Chinese Herbal Medicine in Controlled Clinical Trials

One of the four studies, with 47 participants (H105), assessed the safety of CHM for depression. Nausea (2 cases) and diarrhea (2 cases) were reported in participants using CHM, while 25 AEs were reported in the fluoxetine group including dry mouth (5 cases), insomnia (4 cases), nausea (4 cases), anxiety (3 cases), tiredness (3 cases), dizziness (2 cases), headache (2 cases), and constipation (2 cases).

# Non-controlled Studies of Chinese Herbal Medicine

Thirteen non-controlled studies evaluated CHM in 645 participants with depression (H109–H121). Treatment duration ranged from two to 12 weeks. Nine case series (H109–H112, H114–H119) assessed CHM alone, including three studies using extracted CHM capsules (*Yu shen* pills 愈神丸 combined with *Shu gan jie yu* capsules 舒肝解郁胶囊, *Qi shen fu kang* capsules 芪参复康胶囊 and Korean Red Ginseng extract capsules) (H113, H120, H121). Four studies assessed the effect of integrative CHM (H110, H114, H117, H118) including two studies that used a combination of CHM and antidepressants (H110, H114), and two that used CHM and psychotherapy (H117, H118).

Thirteen formulae (11 named and 2 unnamed) were studied. The most commonly used formula was *Chai hu shu gan san* 柴胡疏肝散, used in five studies including two modified versions (H109, H111, H112, H118, H119). One study used individualised syndrome differentiation and treatment (H109). Fifty-seven herbs were used in the formulae and the most common were *chai hu* 柴胡, *bai shao* 白芍, *fu ling* 茯苓, *gan cao* 甘草, *yu jin* 郁金, *suan zao ren* 酸枣仁, and *xiang fu* 香附.

### Safety of Chinese Herbal Medicine in Non-controlled Studies

Only two studies reported AEs (H114, H121). Adverse events after taking modified *Dan zhi xiao yao san* 丹栀逍遥散加减 and fluoxetine included dry mouth (10 cases), constipation (4 cases), blurred vision (2 cases), dizziness (1 case), electrocardiogram changes (1 case), and elevated aminotransferases (1 case) (H114). Sixteen cases of AEs were reported after taking Korean Red Ginseng extract capsules, including gastrointestinal upset (5 cases), headache (4 cases), insomnia (3 cases), hypersomnia (2 cases), and hair loss (2 cases) (H121).

## Clinical Evidence for Commonly Used Chinese Herbal Medicine Treatments

Eighteen studies (H23, H31, H34, H35, H46, H50, H51, H58, H67, H74, H76, H80, H84, H89, H93, H95, H102, H103) evaluated six formulae recommended in the clinical practice guidelines and textbooks referred to in Chapter 2. These included *Xiao yao san (wan)* 逍遥散(丸), *Chai hu shu gan san* 柴胡疏肝散, *Dan zhi xiao yao san* 丹栀逍遥散, *Ban xia hou po tang* 半夏厚朴汤, *Gui pi tang* 归脾汤, and *Yue ju wan* 越鞠丸. Evidence for *Xiao yao san (wan)* 逍遥散(丸) (H50, H74, H80, H103), *Chai hu shu gan san* 柴胡疏肝散 (H46, H58, H89), and *Dan zhi xiao yao san* 丹栀逍遥散 (H34, H35, H51) have been reported in the previous section of RCT evidence for individual formulae. *Ban xia hou po tang* 半夏厚朴汤, *Gui pi tang* 归脾汤, and *Yue ju wan* 越鞠丸 were evaluated in three studies separately (H31, H95, H102).

### Ban xia hou po tang 半夏厚朴汤

In terms of depression severity measured by HRSD-24, *Ban xia hou po tang* was superior to venlafaxine in one study (n = 70) (MD: –4.29 [–7.11, –1.47]) (H31).

### Gui pi tang 归脾汤

The HRSD-24 was assessed in one study (n = 60) of *Gui pi tang* compared with fluoxetine and it was not superior (MD: –0.17 [–2.34, 2.00]) (H95).

## Yue ju wan 越鞠丸

One study, including 20 participants, compared a combination of *Yue ju wan* and fluoxetine with fluoxetine alone (H102). Efficacy results could not be analysed. A total of four AEs were reported in the integrative medicine group, including two cases each of diarrhea and constipation. Five AEs were reported in the fluoxetine group, including three cases of constipation and two cases of diarrhea.

# Summary of Chinese Herbal Medicine Clinical Evidence

In total, 121 clinical studies evaluated CHM for depression. Randomised controlled trials were the most common study design. Chinese herbal medicine alone, or combined with antidepressants as intervention, and antidepressants as control were the most common. The most common antidepressants were SSRIs. Diagnostic instruments included the Chinese Classification of Mental Disorders (CCMD) (75 studies), Diagnostic and Statistical Manual of Mental Disorders (DSM) (21 studies), and the International Classification of Diseases (ICD) (5 studies). All participants had depression, and a small number had depression subtypes such as postpartum or menopausal depression. Age ranged from 18 to 65 years. Common CM syndromes described in studies were Liver *qi* stagnation, Heart and Spleen deficiency, Liver *qi* stagnation with Spleen deficiency, *qi* stagnation transforming into heat, phlegm stagnation, melancholy disturbing the mind, and Heart and Kidney not interacting. All CHM interventions were orally administrated. Treatment duration ranged from one week to 12 weeks. The commonly used formulae were *Chai hu shu gan san* 柴胡疏肝散 (7 studies), *Dan zhi xiao yao san* 丹栀逍遥散 (4 studies), *Xiao yao san/wan* 逍遥散/丸 (4 studies), *Bu shen shu gan hua yu tang* 补肾疏肝化瘀汤 (2 studies), *An shen ding zhi tang* 安神定志汤 (2 studies), and *Jia wei xiao yao capsules* 加味逍遥胶囊 (2 studies). The three most common herbs were *chai hu* 柴胡, *fu ling/fu shen* 茯苓/茯神, and *shao yao* 芍药.

Depression symptoms were most commonly assessed using the HRSD and other depression severity instruments such as the SDS, the MADRS and the EPDS. Relapse and remission of depression, quality of life, functional capacity, and suicidality were not commonly assessed in the included studies.

## Chinese Herbal Medicine

Chinese herbal medicine was superior to placebo, in terms of reducing depression severity, and participants taking CHM and placebo reported similar AEs. CHM showed significant effects on improving depression and accompanied symptoms, and appeared to be safe. However, the number and size of placebo studies was small.

Chinese herbal medicine showed promising effects when compared with antidepressants, in terms of improving clinical symptoms and alleviating depression severity. Meta-analyses for all depression severity outcome measures indicated consistent results, that is, CHM was superior to antidepressants. However, the majority of studies in the included meta-analyses were judged at "high" risk of bias for blinding of participants, personnel and outcome assessors. In addition, the pooled results showed considerable heterogeneity that could not be explained by subgroup analysis. The reasons for heterogeneity may include variable aetiologies for depression, and different CHM interventions, in terms of treatment duration, dosage, and medication compliance. Chinese herbal medicine showed the largest effect when treatment duration was six weeks or less. This may indicate a strong placebo effect in these participants or the time course and duration of effect is short. Chinese herbal medicine also resulted in more benefit than antidepressants for postpartum depression and menopausal depression.

As for safety, the total AEs in the CHM group was half that of the antidepressants group. The most common AE in the CHM group was dry mouth. The GRADE assessment indicated the evidence was of "low" to "moderate" certainty. Despite the positive results, some caution should be taken in interpreting the findings because studies had methodological shortfalls and there was heterogeneity in the results. Overall, CHM showed promising effects compared with antidepressants and appeared to be safe.

## Integrative Medicine

Chinese herbal medicine combined with antidepressants showed more benefits than antidepressants alone, in terms of reducing depression severity. However, there were methodological shortfalls and studies had unclear sequence generation and allocation concealment, and a lack of blinding of participants and personnel. In addition, the pooled results had considerable heterogeneity, which might be due to inconsistency across studies in terms of depression aetiology, CHM, study protocols, treatment duration, and outcome measurement. The heterogeneity reduced in subgroups of outcome versions. In terms of postpartum depression, CHM plus antidepressants were superior to antidepressants alone. The additional benefit brought by CHM for menopausal depression, compared to antidepressants, remained uncertain as there was only one study with a small sample size. As for effective rate, CHM did not provide additional improvement to antidepressants alone.

The total AEs in the integrative medicine group were less than the antidepressants group. The result should be interpreted cautiously as the number of studies was limited and the comparative effect size was very small. The evidence analysis using the GRADE approach showed studies were of "low" certainty.

CHM combined with psychotherapy, compared to psychotherapy alone, reduced depression symptoms, as did CHM combined with antidepressants and psychotherapy, compared to antidepressants and psychotherapy alone. However, the meta-analyses included studies at "high" risk of bias for blinding of participants, personnel and assessors. The additional benefit brought by integrative medicine, compared to antidepressants and/or psychotherapy, remains uncertain because the study numbers were low and the sample size was small. Overall, the effect of CHM combined with conventional medicine, including antidepressants and psychotherapy, for depression remains uncertain as the evidence is of "low" certainty. However, CHM appears to be safe.

In summary, the best available evidence indicates that CHM can improve depressive symptoms and depression severity and it appears to be safe. A wide range of CHM interventions show promising benefits for people with depression. However, there is no outstanding herb or individual formula that outperforms the others. This is because the number of consistent studies assessing the same CM syndromes and formula over the same period of time are limited. Although the comparative effectiveness between CHM and conventional medicine, such as antidepressants and psychotherapy, remains inconclusive, CHM appears to be well tolerated by people with depression. Until further conclusive evidence is generated, clinical decision-making for people with depression should incorporate their depression aetiology, CM syndrome, treatment preference, and previous experience with antidepressants, psychotherapy, and CHM.

# References

1. Zhao H, Wan X, and Chen JX. (2009) A Mini Review of Traditional Chinese Medicine for the Treatment of Depression in China. *Am J Chinese Med* **37**(2): 207–213.
2. Bulter L and Pilkington K. (2013) Chinese Herbal Medicine and Depression: The Research Evidence. *Evid Based Complement Altern Med* **2013**: 739716.
3. Yeung WF, Chung KF, Ng KY, *et al.* (2014) A systematic review on the efficacy, safety and types of Chinese herbal medicine for depression. *J Psychiatric Res* **57**: 165–175.
4. Yeung WF, Chung KF, Ng KY, *et al.* (2014) A meta-analysis of the efficacy and safety of traditional Chinese medicine formula Ganmai Dazao decoction for depression. *J Ethnopharmacology* **153**: 309–317.
5. Yeung WF, Chung KF, Ng KY, *et al.* (2015) Prescription of Chinese Herbal Medicine in Pattern-Based Traditional Chinese Medicine Treatment for Depression: A Systematic Review. *Evid Based Complement Altern Med* **2015**: 160189.
6. Jun HJ, Choi TY, Lee JA, *et al.* (2014) Herbal medicine (Gan Mai Da Zao decoction) for depression: A systematic review and meta-analysis of randomized controlled trials. *Maturitas* **79**: 370–380.
7. Peng L, Zhang X, Kang DY, *et al.* (2014) Effectiveness and safety of Wuling capsule for post stroke depression: A systematic review. *Complement Ther Med* **22**: 549–566.
8. Ren Y, Zhu CJ, Wu JJ, *et al.* (2015) Comparison between herbal medicine and fluoxetine for depression: A systematic review of randomized controlled trials. *Complement Ther Med* **23**: 674–684.
9. 中医病症诊断疗效标, 国家中医药管理局, 南京: 南京大学出版社, 1995.

**References for Included Chinese Herbal Medicine Clinical Studies**

| Study No. | References |
|---|---|
| H1 | 艾维颖, 高山凤, 阚秀莲, 牛秀梅, 张冲 5. 补血益气组方联合心理干预治疗产后抑郁症的临床研究. 实用药物与临床, 2011, **14**(03): 196–198. |
| H2 | 曹爱群, 郭永林, 张旭桥. 柴胡解郁汤治疗肝郁血虚型抑郁症30例. 中国中医药现代远程教育, 2010, **8**(02): 23. |
| H3 | 曹欣冬, 王伟. "益肾安神解郁汤"配合文拉法辛治疗难治性重度抑郁症38例临床研究. 江苏中医药, 2008, **40**(8): 19–21. |
| H4 | 常耀军. 氟西汀联合中医辨证治疗抑郁症对照研究. 内蒙古中医药, 2013, **32**(14): 25–26. |
| H5 | 陈莉莉. 自拟解郁方联合氟西汀等综合治疗产后抑郁症的临床研究. 中国初级卫生保健, 2015, **29**(12): 94–96. |
| H6 | 陈利平, 吴整军, 王发渭, 段冬梅. 舒郁散治疗抑郁症临床研究. 中国中医急症, 2009, **18**(10): 1583–1584. |
| H7 | 陈琳. 加味逍遥胶囊治疗62例轻中度抑郁症气郁化火证临床疗效观察. 北京中医药大学, 2014. |
| H8 | 陈明伦. 柴桂温胆定志汤治疗精神抑郁症理论研究与临床观察. 北京中医药大学, 2007. |
| H9 | 陈宁红, 王书礼, 王钰. 还少胶囊抗抑郁的临床研究. 南京中医药大学学报, 2010, **26**(06): 471–472. |
| H10 | 陈少玫, 张小丽, 林安基, 冯桂贞. 忘忧方治疗30～50岁抑郁障碍患者的疗效观察. 辽宁中医药大学学报, 2009, **11**(8): 92–94. |
| H11 | 陈伟, 刘磊, 杨雪山, 王妮娜, 刘宗涛. 归脾汤加味联合艾司西酞普兰治疗抑郁症的临床观察. 世界中西医结合杂志, 2013, **8**(08): 829–831. |
| H12 | 陈玉庆. 养血柔肝法治疗产后抑郁症临床观察. 卫生职业教育, 2012, **30**(01): 142. |
| H13 | 陈志彬, 马忠金, 聂凤华. 茯苓神志爽心丸治疗产后抑郁症34例临床观察. 河北中医, 2015, **37**(06): 844–845. |
| H14 | 陈卓, 丁亮吾. 柴胡加龙骨牡蛎汤合百合知母汤治疗抑郁症40例临床观察. 中医临床研究, 2012, **4**(03): 38–39. |
| H15 | 程坤, 颜红, 段可杰. 自拟中药方对抑郁症治疗作用的观察. 中医药临床杂志, 2008(04): 375–376. |
| H16 | 丁志杰. 通络开郁汤合并舍曲林治疗抑郁症的对照研究. 卫生职业教育, 2006(22): 147–148. |
| H17 | 董焘. 加味栀子豉汤治疗抑郁症临床研究. 河南中医, 2016, **36**(05): 867–868. |

**(*Continued*)**

| Study No. | References |
| --- | --- |
| H18 | 董宁, 史付鑫, 崔应麟. 疏肝解郁颗粒配氟西汀治疗肝气郁结型抑郁症30例. 光明中医, 2012, **27**(12): 2515–2516. |
| H19 | 段德香, 王萍. 柴胡解郁汤合马普替林治疗抑郁障碍疗效分析. 中国中医药信息杂志, 2010, **17**(08): 55–56. |
| H20 | 方蓓欢. 调血解郁汤、文拉法辛内服对产后抑郁患者的临床效果观察. 中国中医药科技, 2014, **21**(06): 666–667. |
| H21 | 高楠. 乐心汤治疗围绝经期抑郁症的临床观察. 黑龙江中医药大学, 2010. |
| H22 | 高新立, 马玲, 闫翌君, 马闯胜, 乔建国. 中西医结合治疗抑郁症60例. 河南中医, 2013, **33**(06): 943–944. |
| H23 | 苟汝红, 窦建军, 董江波, 邹永江, 徐德会, 赵长苓. 安神定志方联合度洛西汀治疗抑郁症56例疗效观察. 河北中医, 2015, **37**(10): 1508–1510. |
| H24 | 郭建红, 王顺顺, 范荣. 柴胡疏肝散合甘麦大枣汤加减治疗产后抑郁症的临床观察. 北方药学, 2011, **8**(02): 18–20. |
| H25 | 郭艳青, 苏亚妹. 中西医结合治疗肝气郁结型抑郁症30例. 中医研究, 2010, **23**(07): 46–47. |
| H26 | 何晗, 任丽蓉. 逍遥散加减合氟西汀治疗产后抑郁症临床观察. 湖北中医杂志, 2008, **30**(12): 37–38. |
| H27 | 黄娜娜, 濮欣, 何希俊, 叶沐镕. 温阳解郁汤治疗脾肾阳虚型抑郁症30例. 中医研究, 2014, **27**(08): 25–27. |
| H28 | 霍磊. 礞石滚痰丸加减方对痰热郁结型抑郁症疗效及生活质量影响的临床研究. 山东中医药大学, 2010. |
| H29 | 雷萍萍, 符利文. 中西医结合治疗产后抑郁症疗效观察. 现代中西医结合杂志, 2015, **24**(23): 2582–2583. |
| H30 | 李光义. 加味二仙汤治疗更年期抑郁症的临床研究. 山东中医药大学, 2014. |
| H31 | 李丽娜, 高凌云. 半夏厚朴汤加味治疗躯体症状占优势的抑郁症35例. 福建中医药, 2014, **45**(02): 24–25. |
| H32 | 李淑华, 李巨奇, 李卫青, 马全庆, 廖文生, 禤少敏, 夏洪涛, 赖伟娇. 产后抑郁症护理对策及中医药疗效评价. 中国民族民间医药, 2013, **22**(14): 161–163. |
| H33 | 李宇翅. 越鞠升降汤对轻中度抑郁症患者躯体症状的改善作用. 河北中医, 2014, **36**(11): 1641–1643. |
| H34 | 李玉娟, 罗和春, 钱瑞琴, 赵学英, 信红岭, 毕娟. 丹栀逍遥散对抑郁症患者神经免疫内分泌系统的影响. 中国中西医结合杂志, 2007(03): 197–200. |

(*Continued*)

**(Continued)**

| Study No. | References |
|---|---|
| H35 | 连卓, 吴强, 赵胜楠. 舍曲林联合丹栀逍遥散治疗抑郁症对照研究. 临床心身疾病杂志, 2013, **19**(3): 237–238. |
| H36 | 连卓, 吴强, 赵胜楠. 解郁汤联合米氮平治疗抑郁症随机平行对照研究. 实用中医内科杂志, 2012, **26**(02): 63+65. |
| H37 | 梁文慧, 张丁芳. 健脾疏郁方对抑郁症患者 5-羟色胺影响的研究. 中国民间疗法, 2012, **20**(09): 27–28. |
| H38 | 梁鹦. 逍遥散配合帕罗西汀治疗抑郁症38例. 陕西中医, 2010, **31**(06): 677–678. |
| H39 | 林冰, 夏进. 加味柴胡疏肝散治疗抑郁症临床研究. 新中医, 2011, **43**(08): 36–37. |
| H40 | 林基石, 郭晓玲, 陈家旭, 郭铭隆. 解郁醒脾方治疗肝郁脾虚型抑郁症临床观察. 中华中医药杂志, 2011, **26**(02): 338–340. |
| H41 | 林昱, 杨来启, 杨喜民, 邱财荣, 张彦. 补肾解郁法治疗肾虚肝郁型抑郁症临床疗效观察. 中华中医药学刊, 2013, **31**(10): 2143–2145. |
| H42 | 刘冰. 疏肝解郁安神方治疗中度抑郁发作的临床研究. 河南中医药大学;河南中医学院, 2011. |
| H43 | 刘桂玲. 活力苏口服液联合舍曲林治疗气血亏虚型产后抑郁症. 国际中医中药杂志, 2015, **37**(3): 228–231. |
| H44 | 刘杰, 贾竑晓, 王建琴, 许英, 田金洲, 时晶. 解郁颗粒合并帕罗西汀治疗阴虚内热型难治性抑郁症的疗效观察. 中国中西医结合杂志, 2013, **33**(04): 462–465. |
| H45 | 刘魁. 乌梅丸在肝阳虚抑郁症中的临床应用. 山东中医药大学, 2015. |
| H46 | 刘兰英, 王佩蓉, 顾成宇, 金卫东, 冯斌, 陈炯. 柴胡疏肝散合并文拉法辛对抑郁症肝郁气滞型的随机对照研究. 浙江医学教育, 2012, **11**(05): 51–53. |
| H47 | 刘松山, 陈卫银, 刘福友, 薛洁, 刘远新, 赵艳玲, 孟翠霞, 吉海旺. 可欣舒治疗轻、中度抑郁症(肝郁脾虚证)III期临床试验. 中国新药与临床杂志, 2011, **30**(02): 107–110. |
| H48 | 吕静静. 稳心颗粒联合米氮平对抑郁症及血清NE、5-HT和DA的影响. 河北医科大学, 2012. |
| H49 | 吕小荣, 李凤辉. 解郁宁神汤治疗抑郁症40例. 内蒙古中医药, 2014, **33**(10): 11–12. |
| H50 | 吕志国. 疏肝解郁健脾法治疗抑郁症肝郁脾虚型的临床研究. 长春中医药大学, 2011. |

**(*Continued*)**

| Study No. | References |
|---|---|
| H51 | 罗和春, 钱瑞琴, 赵学英, 毕娟, 信红岭, 蒋学柱, 许珂, 阎少校. 丹栀逍遥散治疗抑郁症的临床疗效观察. 中国中西医结合杂志, **2006**(03): 212–214. |
| H52 | 马菁菁, 林海. 逍遥散合酸枣仁汤加减治疗轻度抑郁症40例. 河南中医, 2011, **31**(09): 1063–1064. |
| H53 | 毛稚霞, 李根起, 杨媛, 郭新宇, 程娟, 张京华. 解郁汤联合氟西汀治疗肝郁脾虚型抑郁症30例临床研究. 河北中医, 2012, **34**(02): 223–226. |
| H54 | 米惠茹, 张跃进, 张炜冉, 高绍芳. 健脾调肝法对产后抑郁症患者汉密尔顿抑郁量表、副反应量表的影响. 河北中医药学报, 2014, **29**(03): 32–33+49. |
| H55 | 潘洪峰, 董湘玉, 刘瑶, 许建阳, 曾强, 梁佳. 越鞠保和丸治疗轻中度抑郁症的临床疗效观察. 时珍国医国药, 2008, **19**(4): 887–889. |
| H56 | 彭卫. 度洛西汀合逍遥膏治疗抑郁症33例临床疗效观察. 中国民间疗法, 2012, **20**(08): 49–50. |
| H57 | 石洲宝, 陈林庆, 刘敏科. "解郁胶囊"治疗抑郁症临床研究. 甘肃中医, 2009, (8): 31–33. |
| H58 | 宋颖民. 疏肝解郁理气法治疗抑郁症30例. 中国中医药现代远程教育, 2011, **9**(16): 7,74. |
| H59 | 孙利, 谷春华, 任君霞, 田野, 杨立波, 张喜芬. 乌灵胶囊治疗轻中度抑郁症的随机对照临床观察. 中国中医基础医学杂志, 2013, **19**(03): 290–291. |
| H60 | 汤久慧, 张丽萍, 吴沛然, 颜红. 加味温胆汤与氟西汀治疗抑郁症的临床对照研究. 环球中医药, 2013, **6**(04): 253–257. |
| H61 | 童梓顺, 刘赟, 徐琰. 帕罗西汀联合加味逍遥散治疗抑郁症的随机对照研究. 四川精神卫生, 2016, **29**(01): 31–34. |
| H62 | 汪显敏, 陈碧, 王东. 解郁柔肝汤治疗产后抑郁症疗效观察. 中医药导报, 2015, **21**(13): 74–76. |
| H63 | 王丹. 补益心脾法治疗产后抑郁症的临床疗效评价研究. 北京中医药大学, 2012. |
| H64 | 王化宁, 张瑞国, 陈云春, 王怀海, 汪卫东, 谭庆荣. 喜乐宁冲剂治疗抑郁症疗效分析. 实用中医药杂志, 2013, **29**(01): 2–3. |
| H65 | 王军峰. 养阴清肝汤联合帕罗西汀治疗抑郁症躯体化症状研究. 中国民康医学, 2013, **25**(20): 64. |
| H66 | 许二平. 加味丹栀逍遥散胶囊治疗抑郁症的临床和机制研究. 南京中医药大学, 2007. |
| H67 | 许凤全, 张莹, 张琳园. 补肾疏肝化瘀汤治疗围绝经期抑郁症82例临床研究. 河北中医, 2013, **35**(03): 333–334. |

*(Continued)*

**(*Continued*)**

| Study No. | References |
|---|---|
| H68 | 杨红娜, 王骞, 姜琳, 乔晶. 保神汤合氟西汀治疗抑郁症的临床研究. 中医药学报, 2010, **38**(05): 108–110. |
| H69 | 杨仁旭, 董艳, 王东梅. 舒解乐无糖颗粒治疗抑郁症的临床研究. 中华医药荟萃, 2002, **01**(5): 16–17. |
| H70 | 杨森, 刘东义. 二合逍遥汤联合氟西汀治疗抑郁症临床观察. 四川中医, 2012, **30**(05): 77–78. |
| H71 | 姚丽娟, 顾钟忠, 嵇冰, 艾宗耀, 沈鑫华, 刘坚白. 郁消Ⅰ号治疗肝气郁结型抑郁症的临床观察. 中国中医药科技, 2014, **21**(05): 546–547. |
| H72 | 叶青, 蔡定芳, 周洁, 顾超, 袁灿兴. 镇惊定志合剂治疗轻中度抑郁症的临床研究. 辽宁中医杂志, 2015, **42**(09): 1686–1688. |
| H73 | 易正辉, 朱丽萍, 龙彬, 姚培芬, 赵根祥, 沈阿珍, 吴国君, 吴海苏, 张六平, 汪作为, 伍毅. 帕罗西汀合并柴胡逍遥合剂治疗抑郁症的临床观察. 中国中西医结合杂志, 2010, **30**(12): 1257–1260. |
| H74 | 尹钰荣, 吴莉娜, 张淼. 盐酸氟西汀配合中成药治疗孕中期引产产妇产后抑郁的研究. 临床和实验医学杂志, 2011, **10**(19): 1513–1515. |
| H75 | 于学平, 张鑫, 刘晓莹. 理气化痰法治疗抑郁症临床观察. 辽宁中医杂志, 2013, **40**(11): 2292–2293. |
| H76 | 余明, 庚晓, 李凝, 尤红, 刘春梅, 李幼东, 王学义. 安神定志汤联合舍曲林治疗抑郁症对照研究. 河北医药, 2011, **33**(13): 2054–2055. |
| H77 | 臧慧莉. "舒郁方"治疗女性更年期抑郁症的临床及实验研究. 南京中医药大学, 2008. |
| H78 | 张广强, 张广普, 艾长明, 谢永强, 赵文学, 岳春芝. 枣仁补血汤联合氟西汀治疗更年期抑郁症38例临床观察. 北京中医药, 2009, **28**(11): 873–874. |
| H79 | 张光茹, 孙巧, 王界成, 宫圣, 王志华, 李玉华. 解郁合欢汤治疗抑郁症的临床观察. 青海医药杂志, 2009, **39**(08): 84–85. |
| H80 | 张华东, 苏慧. 帕罗西汀加逍遥丸治疗抑郁症的临床对照研究. 现代中西医结合杂志, 2009, **18**(33): 4060–4061+4063. |
| H81 | 张静, 汤庆平, 徐伟杰. 中药辅助舍曲林治疗抑郁症的疗效观察. 中华中医药学刊, 2014, **32**(11): 2800–2802. |
| H82 | 张龙生. 柴胡龙骨牡蛎汤加减治疗抑郁障碍临床观察. 河北医药, 2010, **32**(22): 3185–3186. |
| H83 | 张培智. 金香疏肝片治疗抑郁症(肝郁脾虚证)的随机双盲双模拟多中心平行对照研究. 世界临床药物, 2014, **35**(07): 399–403+416. |

**(*Continued*)**

| Study No. | References |
|---|---|
| H84 | 张莹. 补肾疏肝化瘀方治疗肾虚肝郁型女性更年期抑郁症的临床研究. 北京中医药大学, 2013. |
| H85 | 张瑜, 李向丽, 彭晓明. 抗抑郁药配合小柴胡汤治疗抑郁症临床观察. 中华实用中西医杂志, 2004, **17**(7): 1017–1018. |
| H86 | 张志全. 郁乐疏合剂治疗抑郁症(肝郁化火证)的随机对照研究. 成都中医药大学, 2009. |
| H87 | 张子梅, 王云, 冯砚国, 孙富根, 刘金喜. 中西医结合治疗抑郁症36例. 医药导报, 2009, **28**(10): 1279–1280. |
| H88 | 赵海梅, 姜红, 庞铁良. 柴桂开郁汤治疗肝郁痰阻型抑郁症38例临床研究. 河北中医, 2016, **38**(02): 209–211. |
| H89 | 赵雪萍, 林汉. 氟西汀联用柴胡疏肝散加味治疗产后抑郁症. 辽宁中医杂志, 2006, **33**(5): 586–587. |
| H90 | 钟磊. 自拟开郁宁神汤治疗抑郁症的临床观察. 光明中医, 2013, **28**(05): 931–932. |
| H91 | 钟向阳, 李秋琼, 缪雪娜. 自拟柴胡加龙骨牡蛎汤加减治疗抑郁症50例. 中国保健营养(下旬刊), 2012,(11): 4746–4747. |
| H92 | 周博, 颜红. 中西医结合治疗肝郁脾虚型抑郁症30例临床疗效观察. 天津中医药, 2012, **29**(04): 329–331. |
| H93 | 周杰. 加味逍遥胶囊治疗轻中度抑郁症气郁化火证多中心随机对照临床研究. 中国中医科学院, 2013. |
| H94 | 周梦煜. 疏肝解郁汤联合西酞普兰治疗抑郁症40例. 中医研究, 2012, **25**(03): 33–34. |
| H95 | 朱晨军, 李侠, 曲淼. 归脾汤治疗心脾两虚型抑郁症30例. 中国实验方剂学杂志, 2014, **20**(16): 209–213. |
| H96 | 朱晶萍. 酸枣仁汤加减治疗产后抑郁症疗效观察. 新中医, 2014, **46**(07): 105–106. |
| H97 | 宗成翠. 益肾清心汤治疗抑郁症的临床研究. 山东中医药大学, 2014. |
| H98 | Akhondzadeh S, Kashani L, Fotouhi, A, *et al.* (2003). Comparison of Lavandula angustifolia Mill. tincture and imipramine in the treatment of mild to moderate depression: a double-blind, randomized trial. *Prog Neuropsychopharmacol Biol Psychiatry* **27**(1): 123–127. |
| H99 | Akhondzadeh S, Fallah-Pour H, Afkham, K, Jamshidi, AH and Khalighi-Cigaroudi, F. (2004). Comparison of Crocus sativus L. and imipramine in the treatment of mild to moderate depression: a pilot double-blind randomized trial [ISRCTN45683816]. *BMC Complement Altern Med* **4**: 12. |

*(Continued)*

**(*Continued*)**

| Study No. | References |
| --- | --- |
| H100 | Akhondzadeh S, Tahmacebi-Pour N, Noorbala, A A *et al.* (2005). Crocus sativus L. in the treatment of mild to moderate depression: a double-blind, randomized and placebo-controlled trial. *Phytotherapy Res* **19**(2): 148–151. |
| H101 | Akhondzadeh Basti A, Moshiri E, Noorbala, AA *et al.* (2007). Comparison of petal of Crocus sativus L. and fluoxetine in the treatment of depressed outpatients: a pilot double-blind randomized trial. *Prog Neuropsychopharmacol Biol Psychiatry* **31**(2): 439–442. |
| H102 | Wu R, Zhu D, Xia Y, *et al.* (2015). A role of Yueju in fast-onset antidepressant action on major depressive disorder and serum BDNF expression: a randomly double-blind, fluoxetine-adjunct, placebo-controlled, pilot clinical study. *Neuropsychiatr Dis Treat* **11**: 2013–2021. |
| H103 | 徐峰. 逍遥散配合针灸治疗产后抑郁症的临床研究. 世界中西医结合杂志, 2013, **8**(09): 896–899. |
| H104 | 许芳, 唐启盛, 李小黎. 益肾调气法治疗产后抑郁症的随机对照临床研究. 北京中医药, 2013, **32**(03): 200–203. |
| H105 | 郭悟振. 甘麦大枣汤合柴胡加龙骨牡蛎汤治疗抑郁症的研究. 南京中医药大学, 2008. |
| H106 | 王鹏. 孙玉信教授应用柴桂汤治疗郁证(抑郁症)临床观察. 河南中医药大学; 河南中医学院, 2013. |
| H107 | 尚红梅. 中西医结合治疗产后抑郁症的临床疗效. 中国医学工程, 2012, **20**(11): 63–65. |
| H108 | Hemmeter U, Annen B, Bischof R, *et al.* (2001). Polysomnographic effects of adjuvant ginkgo biloba therapy in patients with major depression medicated with trimipramine. *Pharmacopsychiatry* **34**(2): 50–59. |
| H109 | 何谦. 辨证治疗抑郁症65例. 实用中医药杂志, 2012, **28**(06): 465. |
| H110 | 侯振方. 中西医结合治疗抑郁症36例临床观察. 河南中医, 2005, (10): 67–68. |
| H111 | 黄佩珊. 加减柴胡疏肝散联合抗抑郁药物治疗抑郁症68例. 陕西中医, 2012, **33**(06): 666–667. |
| H112 | 贾晓静. 柴胡疏肝散治疗抑郁症35例临床观察. 实用中医内科杂志, 2015, **29**(11): 32–34. |
| H113 | 李东海. 愈神丸联合疏肝解郁胶囊治疗抑郁症疗效观察. 光明中医, 2014, **29**(06): 1227–1228. |
| H114 | 林立. 中西医结合治疗抑郁症的临床分析. 中国当代医药, 2009, **16**(18): 176–177. |

**(*Continued*)**

| Study No. | References |
|---|---|
| H115 | 鲁晶, 毛丽军, 边薇. 周绍华疏肝解郁经验方治疗肝郁气滞型抑郁症临床观察. 辽宁中医杂志, 2011, **38**(10): 2024–2026. |
| H116 | 曲亚楠. 自拟解郁安神汤治疗抑郁症80例疗效观察. 中国民间疗法, 2014, **22**(09): 35–36. |
| H117 | 沈莉, 颜红. 祛湿化痰法治疗抑郁症33例. 新中医, 2007, **39**(7): 66–67. |
| H118 | 尉志军. 柴胡疏肝散加味配合心理治疗抑郁症35例. 中国医院用药评价与分析, 2007, **7**(5): 379–380. |
| H119 | 余波, 李军. 柴胡舒肝散加味治疗抑郁症36例. 现代中医药, 2008, **28**(5): 14–15. |
| H120 | 赵瑾, 贾婷, 吴兴曲, 杨来启, 李新田, 戴捷, 李亚萍. 芪参复康胶囊治疗抑郁症的临床疗效观察. 中国健康心理学杂志, 2013, **21**(06): 830–831. |
| H121 | Jeong HG, Ko YH, Oh SY, *et al*. (2015). Effect of Korean Red Ginseng as an adjuvant treatment for women with residual symptoms of major depression. *Asia Pac Psychiatry* **7**(3): 330–336. |

# 6

# Pharmacological Actions of Frequently Used Herbs

## OVERVIEW

The available experimental evidence of herbs from the most frequently reported herbs used in randomised controlled trials were reviewed. Many herbal extracts showed antidepressant activities in animal models of depression. Underlying mechanisms such as neurogenesis, anti-oxidant and regulation of the hypothalamic-pituitary-adrenal axis are reported, elucidating possible mechanisms for the antidepressant activities of herbal and formula extracts.

## Introduction

This chapter includes the preclinical evidence available for the frequently used herbs identified in randomised controlled trials (RCTs) for depression. Despite the common use of the herbs in clinical studies, experimental studies of Chinese herbal medicine (CHM) in cell and animal models, relevant to depression, were limited. We were able to identify and review experimental data for the following herbs: *Chai hu* 柴胡, *shao yao* 芍药, *gan cao* 甘草, *yuan zhi* 远志, *shi chang pu* 石菖蒲, *zhi ke* 枳壳, *di huang* 地黄, and *dan shen* 丹参. *Xiao yao san* 逍遥散 and *Chai hu shu gan san* 柴胡舒肝散 were the most frequently studied formula in RCTs for depression, therefore, experimental evidence was reviewed for these formulae.

There are several experimental animal models that aim to mimic the human experience of depression. Herbs and formulae have been tested for their antidepressive functions in these models. In the forced swim test, rats swim in a situation of stress. The test reflects a measure of behavioural despair.[1,2] The forced swim test involves the exposure of the animals to stress which may induce a depressed state.[3]

In the chronic unpredictable stress model, the animals exhibit an increased hypothalamic-pituitary-adrenal (HPA) axis sensitivity and a decrease in responses to pleasant stimuli such as a sweet solution.[4] Some studies refer to this as the chronic unpredictable mild stress or chronic mild stress model. The tail suspension test is used for assessing antidepressant-like activity in mice.[5] The test is based on the fact that animals subjected to the short-term stress, will develop an immobile posture.[6]

# Methods

This chapter provides a general overview of the experimental evidence relating to the pharmacology of herbs and their constituent compounds for depression. The constituent compounds were identified by searching herbal monographs, high quality reviews of CHM, herbal medicine encyclopedia,[7] Materia Medica,[8] and/or PubMed. To identify preclinical publications a literature search of PubMed and China National Knowledge Infrastructure (CNKI) was undertaken. The search strategy included the terms for each herb and their constituent compounds. Relevant data were extracted and a summary of the findings reported here.

## Experimental Studies on *chai hu*

*Chai hu* 柴胡 (*Radix Bupleuri*) is derived from the dried root *Bupleurum chinense* DC. var. *scorzonerifolium* Willd. Approximately 74 compounds have been isolated, including essential oils, triterpenoid saponins, polyacetylenes, flavonoids, lignans, fatty acids, and sterols.[9] Triterpenoid saponins, flavonoids, and essential oils, which possess multiple pharmacological activities, are considered to be the main active ingredients of *chai hu*.[9] Crude extracts and pure compounds have been extensively studied and exhibit biological functions such as anti-inflammatory, anti-cancer, anti-pyretic, anti-microbial, anti-viral, hepatoprotective, and immunomodulatory effects.[11] Pharmacological effects in relation to depression are reviewed below.

In rat synaptosomes, polyacetylenes isolated from *chai hu* potently inhibited serotonin, norepinephrine, and dopamine reuptake, and exhibited antidepressant activity comparable with, or better than, neurotransmitter specific inhibitors.[10] In 160 hemodialysis patients diagnosed with depression, the treatment group received 1 gram of root powder *chai hu* given in a capsule daily for three months. Serum nerve growth factor (NGF) and serum brain-derived neurotrophic factor (BDNF) levels were significantly higher in the *chai hu* group when compared to control ($p < 0.01$).[11] NGF and BDNF levels play an important role in the growth, differentiation, and maintenance of neurons. Additionally, serum levels of NGF and BDNF were negatively related with Montgomery–Asberg Depression Rating Scale and positively related with scores of Health Survey RAND-36 ($p < 0.01$).[11] These results indicate that *chai hu* had antidepressant effects and improved quality of life in patients with depression. These results show that increasing neurogenesis is the possible mechanism of *chai hu* in ameliorating depression.[11]

*Chai hu* also demonstrates potent antioxidant effects and plays an important role in regulating cell cycle progression during neurogenesis. In neuronal differentiated SH-SY5Y cells, *chai hu* reversed serum deprivation-induced loss of cell viability, reduced formation of reactive oxygen species, superoxide dismutase activity and regulated levels of cell death regulators B-cell lymphoma 2 and Bax(bcl-2-like protein 4).[12] *Chai hu* also reversed the effect of serum deprivation-decreased cell cycle protein (cyclin D1) and tumor suppression protein (phosphorylated retinoblastoma) expression, and increased cell cycle inhibitor p27 expression.[12] These antioxidant and proliferative effects of *chai hu* may contribute to its antidepressant effects.

## Experimental Studies on *shao yao*

*Shao yao* 芍药 (White peony) is mainly derived from the dried root without bark of *Paeonia lactiflora* Pall. Its constituents include monoterpenoid, triterpenoid, flavonoid, phenol, and tannin chemical groups.[13] Its main bioavailable compounds are paeoniflorin, pentagalloylglucose, gallic acid, albiflorin, and benzoic acid, with most being monoterpene glucosides.[13,14] These compounds have been extensively studied and show anti-inflammatory, anti-oxidant, anti-viral, anti-bacterial, anti-fungal, anti-tumor, anti-arthritis, anti-coagulant anti-platelet, and immuno-modulatory activity.[13,14]

Albiflorin, a monoterpene glycoside, is one of the main components of *shao yao*. In the hypothalamus of freely moving rats, microdialysis showed that albiflorin (3.5, 7.0, 14.0 mg/kg) inhibited the uptake of serotonin and norepinephrine, and displayed robust binding affinities for the transporters of both neurotransmitters.[15] Albiflorin at 10 μM showed no significant affinity to a wide array of central nervous system receptors, presenting binding specificity to serotonin and norepinephrine. These results demonstrate that albiflorin is a novel serotonin and norepinephrine reuptake inhibitor with high selectivity, suggesting its potential as an antidepressant agent.[15]

In mice subjected to the forced swim test and tail suspension test, short-term seven-day treatment with albiflorin significantly decreased immobility time at doses of 3.5, 7.0 and 14.0 mg/kg, without altering the locomotor activity in the mice.[16] Chronic treatment with albiflorin, at doses of 7.0 and 14.0 mg/kg (once daily for 35 days), restored the sucrose preference in chronic unpredictable stressed rats. In the open-field test, albiflorin significantly increased the number of crossings and rearings in the chronic unpredictable stressed rats at all three doses. Chronic treatment with albiflorin also up-regulated hippocampal BDNF expression, hippocampal serotonin, the serotonin metabolite 5-hydroxyindoleacetic acid, and norepinephrine levels of depressed mice.[16]

In mouse models of depression induced using the forced swim test, tail suspension test, and the open field test to exclude false-positive results, *chai hu* and *shao yao* at low, medium, and high doses decreased immobility time in both the forced swim test and tail suspension test. Pre-treatment of the herb pair significantly elevated the concentrations of serotonin and norepinephrine in the hippocampal and cortical tissues after the antipsychotic drug reserpine was administered. The results suggest that *chai hu* and *shao yao* together have antidepressant-like effects. The possible mechanisms of action are through the regulation of the central monoaminergic neurotransmitter system in the hippocampal and cortical tissues.[17]

# Experimental studies on *gan cao*

*Gan cao* 甘草 is derived from the dried roots and rhizomes of *Glycyrrhiza uralensis* Fisch. var. *inflata* Bat. var. *glabra* L. The main bioactive constituents of *gan cao* are triterpenes, saponins, and various types of flavonoids.[8,18] Previous studies have shown that *gan cao* has anti-ulceric, anti-inflammatory, anti-spasmodic, anti-oxidative, anti-allergic, anti-viral, anti-diabetic, anti-cancer, anti-depressive, hepatoprotective, expectorant, and memory enhancing activities.[18]

Liquiritin is a flavone compound from *gan cao*. In a rat model of chronic variable stress-induced depression, daily administration of liquiritin for three weeks effectively reversed alterations in immobility time and sucrose consumption but did not show significant effect on open-field activity. Liquiritin also demonstrated anti-oxidant properties through increased erythrocyte superoxide dismutase activity, inhibition of lipid peroxidation, and reduced production of plasma malondialdehyde, while the antidepressant fluoxetine did not. These results suggest that the antidepressant effects of liquiritin may be related to its anti-oxidant activities.[19]

Total flavonoids extract from *gan cao* (30, 100, 300 mg/kg) were administered to adult rats in a chronic unpredictable stress model of depression.[20] After chronic treatment for 28 days, the flavonoids showed antidepressant functions by increasing the sum of line crosses and number of rears, and decreased the number of fecal boli produced in the open field test. The flavonoids also decreased the immobility time in the forced swim test, as well as in the tail suspension test. In addition, a higher concentration of flavonoids (300 mg/kg) decreased serum corticosterone levels, a marker for stress in rodents. It also increased cell proliferation via hippocampal neurogenesis, indicated by an increased number of new born bromodeoxyuridine positive progenitor cells at the subgranular zone of dentate gyrus region in the hippocampus, suggesting a neurogenesis protective effect.[20]

## Experimental Studies on *yuan zhi*

*Yuan zhi* 远志, the dried root of *Polygala tenuifolia* Willd., is mainly comprised of xanthone, xanthone C-glycosides, triterpene saponins, sucroseesters, and oligosaccharide esters.[21] *Yuan zhi* and its extracts have shown anti-oxidant, anti-inflammatory, cognitive enhancing, and cerebral protecting functions.[22–24]

Antidepressant effects of triterpenoid saponin components derived from *yuan zhi* (Yuanzhi-1 to Yuanzhi-6) were tested in receptor binding assays and behavioral animal models. Yuanzhi-1, -3, -5 and -6 showed antidepressant-like activity in the tail suspension test and forced swim test in mice.[25] The authors highlighted that the effective dose of Yuanzhi-1 (2.5 mg/kg) was lower than the commonly used antidepressant duloxetine (5 mg/kg), and the median lethal dose was similar to duloxetine demonstrating potential clinical efficacy and safety.[25] Yuanzhi-1 also showed a high affinity for the neurotransmitter transporters for serotonin, norepinephrine, and dopamine. These results suggest the potential antidepressant effects of Yuanzhi-1 to Yuanzhi-6.

An active fraction obtained from *yuan zhi* called YZ-50 was assessed in a chronic mild stress depression rat model. Administration of YZ-50 reversed the depression model-induced changes in sucrose consumption, plasma corticosterone levels and open field activity.[26] Rats given YZ-50 also showed reduced effects of chronic mild stress on mood and behaviour. It was thought that the antidepressant properties of YZ-50 were likely mediated by neuroendocrine and neuroprotective systems, with the HPA axis also playing an important role in this process.[26]

In 8-week-old male C54Bl/6 mice, 30 minutes after a single oral administration of *yuan zhi* extract (0.1 mg/kg), antidepressant-like effects were observed and included a decrease in behavioural despair in both the forced swim and tail suspension tests.[27] Two doses of *yuan zhi* extract increased pleasure in rodents exposed to chronic stress, in contrast monoaminergic antidepressants required many repeat doses.[27] On a cellular level, in the hippocampus *yuan zhi* extract modulated glutamatergic synapses in the critical brain circuits involved in depression, and showed the potential of rapid-onset anti-depressant effects.[27]

Three, 6'-disinapoyl sucrose (DISS), is an active oligosaccharide ester component from the root of *yuan zhi*.[28] In rats that have depression induced by chronic mild stress, brain monoamine oxidase (MAO)-A and MAO-B (enzymes that break down neurotransmitters and lead to decreased levels of neurotransmitters), plasma cortisol levels and malondialdehyde (a marker for oxidative stress) levels were increased, while superoxide dismutase antioxidant activity was decreased following chronic mild stress exposures. DISS significantly inhibited MAO-A and MAO-B activity and blocked plasma elevated cortisol levels, an indicator of activation of the HPA axis. In addition, DISS can increase superoxide dismutase anti-oxidant activity, inhibit lipid peroxidation, and lessen production of malondialdehyde, showing anti-oxidant properties.[28]

Another study, using the *yuan zhi* extract DISS for 28 days in chronic mild stress rats, showed improved reward reaction, as measured by increased sucrose consumption.[29] Biologic observations of serum cortisol, hormones and receptor mRNA, indicated that DISS can modulate the HPA axis.[29] It also reversed stress-induced alterations in sucrose consumption and increased mRNA and protein levels in the hippocampus of noradrenergic-regulated plasticity genes and BDNF.[30] Taken together, DISS may possess potent and rapid antidepressant properties, which are mediated via brain enzyme activity, the HPA axis and oxidative systems, and regulation of hippocampus noradrenergic-regulated plasticity genes and neurotrophic factors.

## Experimental Studies on *shi chang pu*

*Shi chang pu* 石菖蒲 is the dried rhizome of *Acorus tatarinowii* Schott. Its main constituents include volatile oils such as α-, β-, γ-asarone, amino acids, and sugars.[8] Volatile oils are considered to be the active ingredients in *shi chang pu* and asarone accounts for more than 90%

of total volatile oil.[31] Alpha-asarone and β-asarone have shown anti-epileptic, anxiolytic, neuroprotective, and hypolipidemic activities.[32]

In forced swim and tail suspension tests, the immobility time of rats is reduced significantly by α-asarone and β-asarone at doses of 20 and 120 mg/kg.[33] In the mouse depression model of tail suspension test, acute treatment with α-asarone showed biphasic action of anti-depressant-like effects at relatively low doses (15 and 20 mg/kg, i.p.) and depressive-like activity at higher doses (50 and 100 mg/kg, i.p.). The antidepressant actions are reversed by pre-treatment of antago-nists of α-1 and α-2 adrenoceptors and serotonin $1_A$ receptors, suggesting that the antidepressant-like effect of α-asarone could be mediated through both noradrenergic (α1 and α2 adrenoceptors) and serotonergic (particularly serotonin $1_A$ receptors) systems.[34]

In the chronic unpredictable mild stress rat model, β-asarone treat-ment partially reversed the depression-like behaviors in both the forced swim and sucrose preference tests. Further analysis showed increased hippocampal neurogenesis, as indicated by bromodeoxyuridine immune-reactivity, and increased expression of BDNF at the level of transcription and translation.[35] Chronic unpredictable mild stress caused a significant reduction in extracellular signal-regulated kinases (ERK) 1 and 2 and cAMP response element-binding protein (CREB) phosphorylation, which is an important neuronal mechanism of depression.[35] Importantly β-asarone did not affect non-stressed rats suggesting it works in a stress-dependent manner to block ERK1/2-CREB signaling and has an effect on neurogenesis.[35]

## Experimental Studies on *zhi ke*

*Zhi ke* 枳壳 (Aurantii Fructus) is the dried immature fruit of *Citrus aurantium* Linn.[36] Major known chemical constituent groups of *zhi ke* are volatile oils, flavonoids and alkaloids.[8,37] Previous studies have shown that *zhi ke* has anti-ischemic and anti-nephrolithic properties, as well as gastrointestinal motility regulating functions.[38–40]

*Zhi ke's* constituents, naringin, hesperidin, neohesperidin, and nobiletin have neuroprotective effects on corticosterone-induced neurotoxicity in neuronal differentiated pheochromocytoma PC12 cells in a dose-dependent manner.[37] *Zhi ke* aqueous extracts significantly decreased the immobility time and dose-dependently increased the locomotor activity, compared to vehicle control in rats in the forced swim test.[41] Mice immobility time during the forced swimming and the tail suspension tests were also significantly reduced with *zhi ke* aqueous extract.[37] The *in vitro* and *in vivo* results suggest that *zhi ke* has antidepressant and neuroprotective effects.

## Experimental Studies on *di huang*

*Di huang* 地黄 is the dried root of *Rehmannia glutinosa* Libosch. Identified chemical constituent groups include iridoids and iridoid glycosides, other glycosides, sugars, organic acids, and amino acids.[8] Studies on *di huang* have shown anti-allergy and anti-inflammatory actions *in vivo* and *in vitro*.[42–44]

In the chronic unpredictable mild stress depression model, reduced locomotion in mice was restored by a low dose of steamed roots of *di huang* (2.5 g/kg) but not high dose *shu di huang* 熟地黄 (5 g/kg).[47] Chronic unpredictable mild stress induction resulted in aggravated gastric ulceration, elevated liver malondialdehyde, reduced total anti-oxidant capability, glutathione content, and superoxide dismutase and catalase activities. *Shu di huang* also improved anti-oxidant activities in mice in a dose-dependent manner.[45] The results produced are similar to those of the antidepressant drug clomipramine.[45] *Shu di huang* has shown to have anti-oxidant and antidepressant functions.

## Experimental Studies on *dan shen*

*Dan shen* 丹参 is from the root of the plant *Salvia miltiorrhiza* Bge. Major known chemical constituents are the quinones, diterpene ketones, diterpene lactones, phenols, and others such as baicalin.[8] Actions of *dan shen* include anti-oxidant, anti-hyperlipidemic, and anti-cancer properties.[46]

Salvianolic acids are bioactive and abundant compounds found in *dan shen*.[47] In mice tested in forced swim and tail suspension tests, salvianolic acid B reduced the immobility time in both tests whilst locomotion in spontaneous motor activity was unchanged.[48,49] Salvianolic acid B also reversed the reduced sucrose preference ratio indicating improved mood.[49] Salvianolic acid B can also improve the imbalance between pro- and anti-inflammatory cytokines in the hippocampus and cortex of chronic mild stress-treated mice.[49] These effects were not observed in the imipramine drug group. Salvianolic acid B also significantly decreased chronic mild stress-induced apoptosis and microglia activation in the hippocampus and cortex, whereas the antidepressant imipramine did not.[49] Salvianolic acid B has shown antidepressant-like effects in chronic mild stress-induced mouse models of depression, as well as showing anti-oxidant activities and inhibition of microglia-related apoptosis in the hippocampus and cortex.

## Experimental Studies on *Xiao yao san*

*Xiao yao san* 逍遥散 is one of the most frequently used herbal formula in clinical research for depression. Ingredients include: *Chai hu* 柴胡, *dang gui* 当归, *fu ling* 茯苓, *bai zhu* 白术, *bo he* 薄荷, *sheng jiang* 生姜, and *gan cao* 甘草.

In mice exposed to interferon-α-induced depression, decreased sucrose consumption and immobility in the forced swim and tail suspension tests was improved significantly after *Xiao yao san* or escitalopram treatment. Further, *Xiao yao san* reduced the number of microglia and expression of indoleamine-2,3-dioxygenase 1, which in turn significantly increased expression of serotonin in the mouse dorsal raphe nucleus.[50] In social isolation and chronic unpredictable mild stress-treated rats, *Xiao yao san* extracts ameliorated depressive-like behaviour. Hypothalamic-pituitary-adrenal axis hyperactivity was demonstrated via the upregulated corticosterone and urocortin 2 levels, these were downregulated by *Xiao yao san* extracts. In addition, neuronal cell numbers were improved and Nissl's body increased by *Xiao yao san*.[51] The effect of *Xiao yao san* extract on the locus coeruleus-norepinephrine system was investigated in chronic immobilisation stress-induced rats. Serum norepinephrine concentrations and norepinephrine biosynthesis enzymes such as tyrosine hydroxylase, dopamine-$\beta$-hydroxylase, and corticotrophin-releasing-factor in locus coeruleus were significantly increased in the rats. The *Xiao yao san*-treated group displayed a significant decrease in norepinephrine levels and expressions of tyrosine hydroxylase, dopamine-$\beta$-hydroxylase, and corticotrophin-releasing-factor compared to the model group. Suggesting *Xiao yao san* aqueous extract improved depressive-like behaviours in rats through inhibition of neuronal activity in the locus coeruleus.[52] Preclinical studies have shown that *Xiao yao san* may exert its antidepressant activities via several different mechanisms.

## Experimental Studies on *Chai hu shu gan san*

*Chai hu shu gan san* 柴胡舒肝散 is another frequently used herbal formula in clinical research for depression. It consists of *chai hu* 柴胡, *chen pi* 陈皮, *shao yao* 芍药, *gan cao* 甘草, *zhi ke* 枳壳, *chuan xiong* 川芎, and *xiang fu* 香附.

In rats exposed to chronic unpredictable stress, chronic administration of *Chai hu shu gan san* aqueous extract for 14 days or more, at a dose of 5.9 g/kg, reduced depressive-like behaviours such as decreased weight gain, and decreased locomotor activity measured by the open field test. *Chai hu shu gan san* also decreased sucrose consumption, with results comparable to the antidepressant drug fluoxetine.[53-55] In chronic unpredictable mild stress-induced rats, the hippocampus ERK5 activation was significantly suppressed and *Chai hu shu gan san* aqueous extracts reversed the stress-induced disruption of ERK5 activity.[54] Decreased levels of phospho-ERK1/2 (P-ERK1/2) and the ratio of P-ERK1/2 to total ERK1/2 in the hippocampus were observed in chronic unpredictable mild stress-induced rats. This was alleviated by chronic administration of *Chai hu shu gan san* aqueous extracts.[55] C-jun amino-terminal kinase signal transduction plays a key role in the apoptosis of nerve cells. *Chai hu shu gan san* aqueous extracts inhibited the expressions of c-jun amino-terminal kinase in the hippocampus in chronic unpredictable mild stress-induced rats.[53] These studies show that *Chai hu shu gan san* exhibits its antidepressant activities through multiple pathways and targets.

## Summary of Pharmacological Actions

In animal models that reflect depression, CHM and their constituent compounds have shown marked antidepressant activities. Some studies suggest neuroendocrine and neurotransmitter-modulatory properties, in addition to anti-oxidant effects. These mechanisms may be the underlying reason of their antidepressant activities. Current experimental evidence suggests that an array of herbal compounds exhibit their antidepressant activities via multiple pathways and targets. Further investigation of key compounds or compound combinations in neuronal cells or depressive animal models are required to further elucidate the possible mechanism of action of CHM for depression.

## References

1. Porsolt RD, Anton G, Blavet N, *et al.* (1978) Behavioural despair in rats: a new model sensitive to antidepressant treatments. *Eur J Pharmacol* **47**(4): 379–391.
2. Porsolt RD, Le Pichon M and Jalfre M. (1977) Depression: a new animal model sensitive to antidepressant treatments. *Nature.* **266**(5604): 730–732.
3. Yankelevitch-Yahav R, Franko M, Huly A, *et al.* (2015) The forced swim test as a model of depressive-like behavior. *J Vis Exp* (97): e52587.
4. Willner P, Wilkes M and Orwin A. (1990) Attributional style and perceived stress in endogenous and reactive depression. *J Affect Disord* **18**(4): 281–287.
5. Steru L, Chermat R, Thierry B, *et al.* (1985) The tail suspension test: a new method for screening antidepressants in mice. *Psychopharmacology* **85**(3): 367–370.
6. Cryan JF, Mombereau C and Vassout A. (2005) The tail suspension test as a model for assessing antidepressant activity: review of pharmacological and genetic studies in mice. *Neurosci Biobehav Rev* **29**(4–5): 571–625.
7. Zhou J, Xie G and Yan X. (2011). Encyclopedia of Traditional Chinese Medicine: Molecular structures, pharmacological activities, natural sources and applications. Berlin: Springer.

8. Bensky D, Clavey S and Stoger E. (2004). Chinese herbal medicine Materia Medica. 3rd ed. Seattle, US: Eastland Press, Inc.

9. Yang F, Dong X, Yin X, *et al.* (2017) Radix Bupleuri: A Review of Traditional Uses, Botany, Phytochemistry, Pharmacology, and Toxicology. *Biomed Res Int* **2017**: 7597596.

10. Liu J, Fang Y, Yang L, *et al.* (2015) A qualitative, and quantitative determination and pharmacokinetic study of four polyacetylenes from Radix Bupleuri by UPLC-PDA-MS. *J Pharm Biomed Anal* **111**: 257–265.

11. Wang X, Feng Q, Xiao Y, *et al.* (2015) Radix Bupleuri ameliorates depression by increasing nerve growth factor and brain-derived neurotrophic factor. *Int J Clin Exp Med* **8**(6): 9205–9217.

12. Seo MK, Cho HY, Lee CH, *et al.* (2013) Antioxidant and Proliferative Activities of Bupleuri Radix Extract Against Serum Deprivation in SH-SY5Y Cells. *Psychiatry Investig* **10**(1): 81–88.

13. Parker S, May B, Zhang C, *et al.* (2016) A Pharmacological Review of Bioactive Constituents of Paeonia lactiflora Pallas and Paeonia veitchii Lynch. *Phytother Res* **30**(9): 1445–1473.

14. He DY and Dai SM. (2011) Anti-inflammatory and immunomodulatory effects of paeonia lactiflora pall., a traditional chinese herbal medicine. *Front Pharmacol* **2**: 10.

15. Jin ZL, Gao N, Xu W, *et al.* (2016) Receptor and transporter binding and activity profiles of albiflorin extracted from Radix paeoniae Alba. *Sci Rep* **6**: 33793.

16. Wang YL, Wang JX, Hu XX, *et al.* (2016) Antidepressant-like effects of albiflorin extracted from Radix paeoniae Alba. *J Ethnopharmacol* **179**: 9–15.

17. Wang Y, Gao SM, Li R, *et al.* (2016) Antidepressant-like effects of the Radix Bupleuri and Radix Paeoniae Alba drug pair. *Neurosci Lett* **633**: 14–20.

18. Zhang Q and Ye M. (2009) Chemical analysis of the Chinese herbal medicine Gan-Cao (licorice). *J Chromatogr A* **1216**(11): 1954–1969.

19. Zhao Z, Wang W, Guo H, *et al.* (2008) Antidepressant-like effect of liquiritin from Glycyrrhiza uralensis in chronic variable stress induced depression model rats. *Behav Brain Res* **194**(1): 108–113.

20. Fan ZZ, Zhao WH, Guo J, *et al.* (2012) [Antidepressant activities of flavonoids from Glycyrrhiza uralensis and its neurogenesis protective effect in rats]. *Yao Xue Xue Bao* **47**(12): 1612–1617.

21. Ling Y, Li Z, Chen M, *et al.* (2013) Analysis and detection of the chemical constituents of Radix Polygalae and their metabolites in rats after oral administration by ultra high-performance liquid chromatography

coupled with electrospray ionization quadrupole time-of-flight tandem mass spectrometry. *J Pharm Biomed Anal* **85**: 1–13.

22. Cheong MH, Lee SR, Yoo HS, *et al.* (2011) Anti-inflammatory effects of Polygala tenuifolia root through inhibition of NF-κB activation in lipopolysaccharide-induced BV2 microglial cells. *J Ethnopharmacol* **137**(3): 1402–1408.

23. Cho N, Huh J, Yang H, *et al.* (2012) Chemical constituents of Polygala tenuifolia roots and their inhibitory activity on lipopolysaccharide-induced nitric oxide production in BV2 microglia. *J Enzyme Inhib Med Chem* **27**(1): 1–4.

24. Ikeya Y, Takeda S, Tunakawa M, *et al.* (2004) Cognitive improving and cerebral protective effects of acylated oligosaccharides in Polygala tenuifolia. *Biol Pharm Bull* **27**(7): 1081–1085.

25. Jin ZL, Gao N, Zhang JR, *et al.* (2014) The discovery of Yuanzhi-1, a triterpenoid saponin derived from the traditional Chinese medicine, has antidepressant-like activity. *Prog Neuropsychopharmacol Biol Psychiatry* **53**: 9–14.

26. Hu Y, Liu P, Guo DH, *et al.* (2010) Antidepressant effects of the extract YZ-50 from Polygala tenuifolia in chronic mild stress treated rats and its possible mechanisms. *Pharm Biol* **48**(7): 794–800.

27. Shin IJ, Son SU, Park H, *et al.* (2014) Preclinical evidence of rapid-onset antidepressant-like effect in Radix Polygalae extract. *PLoS One* **9**(2): e88617.

28. Hu Y, Liu M, Liu P, *et al.* (2011) Possible mechanism of the antidepressant effect of 3,6′-disinapoyl sucrose from Polygala tenuifolia Willd. *J Pharm Pharmacol* **63**(6): 869–874.

29. Hu Y, Liao HB, Liu P, *et al.* (2009) A bioactive compound from Polygala tenuifolia regulates efficiency of chronic stress on hypothalamic-pituitary-adrenal axis. *Pharmazie* **64**(9): 605–608.

30. Hu Y, Liao HB, Dai-Hong G, *et al.* (2010) Antidepressant-like effects of 3,6′-disinapoyl sucrose on hippocampal neuronal plasticity and neurotrophic signal pathway in chronically mild stressed rats. *Neurochem Int* **56**(3): 461–465.

31. Lam KYC, Yao P, Wang H, *et al.* (2017) Asarone from Acori Tatarinowii Rhizome prevents oxidative stress-induced cell injury in cultured astrocytes: A signaling triggered by Akt activation. *PLoS One* **12**(6): e0179077.

32. Chellian R, Pandy V and Mohamed Z. (2017) Pharmacology and toxicology of alpha- and beta-Asarone: A review of preclinical evidence. *Phytomedicine* **32**: 41–58.
33. Han P, Han T, Peng W, *et al.* (2013). Antidepressant-like effects of essential oil and asarone, a major essential oil component from the rhizome of Acorus tatarinowii. *Pharm Biol* **51**(5): 589–594.
34. Chellian R, Pandy V and Mohamed Z. (2016) Biphasic Effects of alpha-Asarone on Immobility in the Tail Suspension Test: Evidence for the Involvement of the Noradrenergic and Serotonergic Systems in Its Antidepressant-Like Activity. *Front Pharmacol* **7**: 72.
35. Dong H, Gao Z, Rong H, *et al.* (2014) Beta-asarone reverses chronic unpredictable mild stress-induced depression-like behavior and promotes hippocampal neurogenesis in rats. *Molecules* **19**(5): 5634–5649.
36. Jiang Y, Bai X, Zhu X, *et al.* (2014) The effects of Fructus Aurantii extract on the 5-hydroxytryptamine and vasoactive intestinal peptide contents of the rat gastrointestinal tract. *Pharm Biol* **52**(5): 581–585.
37. Wu M, Zhang H, Zhou C, *et al.* (2015) Identification of the chemical constituents in aqueous extract of Zhi-Qiao and evaluation of its antidepressant effect. *Molecules* **20**(4): 6925–6940.
38. Kang M, Kim JH, Cho C, *et al.* (2007). Anti-ischemic effect of Aurantii Fructus on contractile dysfunction of ischemic and reperfused rat heart. *J Ethnopharmacol* **111**(3): 584–591.
39. Li X, Liang Q, Sun Y, *et al.* (2015) Potential Mechanisms Responsible for the Antinephrolithic Effects of an Aqueous Extract of Fructus Aurantii. *Evid Based Complement Alternat Med* **2015**: 491409.
40. Tan W, Li Y, Wang Y, *et al.* (2017) Anti-coagulative and gastrointestinal motility regulative activities of Fructus Aurantii Immaturus and its effective fractions. *Biomed Pharmacother* **90**: 244–252.
41. Zhang YJ, Huang W, Huang X, *et al.* (2012) Fructus Aurantii induced antidepressant effect via its monoaminergic mechanism and prokinetic action in rat. *Phytomedicine* **19**(12): 1101–1107.
42. Baek GH, Jang YS, Jeong SI, *et al.* (2012) Rehmannia glutinosa suppresses inflammatory responses elicited by advanced glycation end products. *Inflammation* **35**(4): 1232–1241.
43. Han Y, Jung HW, Lee JY, *et al.* (2012) 2,5-dihydroxyacetophenone isolated from Rehmanniae Radix Preparata inhibits inflammatory responses in lipopolysaccharide-stimulated RAW264.7 macrophages. *J Med Food* **15**(6): 505–510.

44. Sung YY, Yoon T, Jang JY, *et al.* (2011) Topical application of Rehmannia glutinosa extract inhibits mite allergen-induced atopic dermatitis in NC/ Nga mice. *J Ethnopharmacol* **134**(1): 37–44.

45. Zhang D, Wen XS, Wang XY, *et al.* (2009) Antidepressant effect of Shudihuang on mice exposed to unpredictable chronic mild stress. *J Ethnopharmacol* **123**(1): 55–60.

46. Su CY, Ming QL, Rahman K, *et al.* (2015) Salvia miltiorrhiza: Traditional medicinal uses, chemistry, and pharmacology. *Chin J Nat Med* **13**(3): 163–182.

47. Ho JH and Hong CY. (2011) Salvianolic acids: small compounds with multiple mechanisms for cardiovascular protection. *J Biomed Sci* **18**: 30.

48. Feng Y, You Z, Yan S, *et al.* (2012) Antidepressant-like effects of salvia-nolic acid B in the mouse forced swim and tail suspension tests. *Life Sci* **90**(25–26): 1010–1014.

49. Zhang JQ, Wu XH, Feng Y, *et al.* (2016) Salvianolic acid B ameliorates depressive-like behaviors in chronic mild stress-treated mice: involvement of the neuroinflammatory pathway. *Acta Pharmacol Sin* **37**(9): 1141–1153.

50. Wang M, Huang W, Gao T, *et al.* (2017) Effects of Xiao Yao San on Interferon-$\alpha$-Induced Depression in Mice. *Brain Res Bull* **139**: 197–202.

51. Zhu X, Xia O, Han W, *et al.* (2014) Xiao Yao San Improves Depressive-Like Behavior in Rats through Modulation of beta-Arrestin 2-Mediated Pathways in Hippocampus. *Evid Based Complement Alternat Med* **2014**: 902516.

52. Ding XF, Zhao XH, Tao Y, *et al.* (2014) Xiao Yao San Improves Depressive-Like Behaviors in Rats with Chronic Immobilization Stress through Modulation of Locus Coeruleus-Norepinephrine System. *Evid Based Complement Alternat Med* **2014**: 605914.

53. Li YH, Zhang CH, Qiu J, *et al.* (2014) Antidepressant-like effects of Chaihu-Shugan-San via SAPK/JNK signal transduction in rat models of depression. *Pharmacogn Mag* **10**(39): 271–277.

54. Qiu J, Hu SY, Zhang CH, *et al.* (2014) The effect of Chaihu-Shugan-San and its components on the expression of ERK5 in the hippocampus of depressed rats. *J Ethnopharmacol* **152**(2): 320–326.

55. Wang S, Hu S, Zhang C, *et al.* (2011). Effect of Chaihu Shugan San and its components on expression of ERK1/2 mRNA in the hippocampus of rats with chronic mild unpredicted stress depression. *Zhong Nan Da Xue Xue Bao Yi Xue Ban* **36**(2): 93–100.

# 7

# Clinical Evidence for Acupuncture and Related Therapies

## OVERVIEW

Acupuncture and related therapies can treat depression. This chapter evaluates 56 published clinical studies investigating acupuncture and related therapies for depression. Forty-eight studies were randomised controlled trials and eight were non-controlled studies. Acupuncture may reduce depression severity and symptoms.

## Introduction

Acupuncture is an integral part of Chinese medicine (CM) and stimulating acupuncture points can correct imbalances of energy and restore health to the body. Methods of stimulating acupuncture points include:

- Acupuncture: Insertion of an acupuncture needle into acupuncture points;
- Electroacupuncture: After insertion of acupuncture needle into acupuncture points, small electric current runs between the needle pair via electrodes connected to the needles;
- Laser: Application of low level laser to acupuncture points;
- Transcutaneous electrical nerve stimulation (TENS): Application of transdermal electrical current to acupuncture points via conducting pads.

Whilst many of these therapies have ancient roots, several have emerged as new techniques in the last century, including electroacupuncture, laser, and TENS.

## Previous Systematic Reviews

Previously a number of systematic reviews evaluated the efficacy of acupuncture and related therapies, either alone or in combination with, conventional therapies for depression. Smith *et al.*, 2010, included 30 trials (2,812 participants) to investigate the efficacy of acupuncture for major depressive disorder, compared to any type of control.[1] Meta-analysis showed insufficient evidence of a consistent beneficial effect from acupuncture, compared with no treatment or sham acupuncture control. Two trials found acupuncture may have an additive benefit when combined with pharmacotherapy, compared to pharmacotherapy alone. Yet the majority of trials comparing manual acupuncture and electroacupuncture with pharmacotherapy found no difference in effect between groups. The results are limited by "high" risk of bias in most of the included studies.

Another review assessed the beneficial effects of acupuncture in patients with depression in 26 randomised controlled trials (RCTs) (2,173 participants).[2] A significant beneficial effect was found for acupuncture, compared to control, measured by the Hamilton Rating Scale for Depression (HRSD). Subgroup analysis showed that electroacupuncture and manual acupuncture have similar effects. The methodological quality of the included studies was "low" and the authors recommended further studies to improve the quality of the evidence. Shen *et al.*, 2014, included 13 studies (884 participants) to investigate the efficacy of acupuncture for depression.[3] Meta-analysis showed that acupuncture was more effective than pharmacotherapy, in terms of improving effective rate. There were no significant differences between the number of adverse events (AEs) in the acupuncture group and pharmacotherapy group. Results should be interpreted with caution due to the methodological short-comings of the included studies. Authors suggest that large scale, multi-centre RCTs should be conducted to produce objective and reliable results.

Zhang *et al.*, 2010, investigated the efficacy of acupuncture alone, or as integrative medicine, for depression. Meta-analysis was conducted using 20 "high"-quality (Jadad score ≥ 3) RCTs.[4] Acupuncture was comparable to antidepressants but there was no evidence that acupuncture combined with antidepressants could yield better outcomes than antidepressants alone. There were fewer AEs in the acupuncture groups, compared to antidepressants. The authors concluded that acupuncture is safe and effective in treating depression and could be considered a treatment option. Chan *et al.*, 2015, investigated the effect of combined acupuncture and antidepressants, compared with antidepressants alone.[5] The review included 13 studies involving 1,046 participants. Meta-analysis showed significant differences in HRSD scores and effective rate in favour of acupuncture combined with selective serotonin reuptake inhibitors (SSRIs).

Zhang *et al.*, 2016, evaluated the efficacy and safety of combined SSRIs and electroacupuncture. Six RCTs (431 participants) were analysed.[6] The meta-analysis revealed that the combined therapy of SSRIs and electroacupuncture was superior to SSRIs alone, in terms of the HRSD, Zung Self-rating Depression Scale (SDS), and side effect rating scales of Asberg (SERS), after one to four weeks of treatment. The authors concluded that the early treatment of primary depression, using both SSRIs and electroacupuncture, is more effective than SSRIs alone.

# Identification and Characteristics of Clinical Studies

A total of 41,942 citations were identified through database searches and 2,218 full-text articles reviewed for eligibility. Fifty-six clinical studies (A1–A56) met the inclusion criteria. Forty-eight studies were RCTs and eight were non-controlled studies; controlled clinical trials (CCTs) were not identified (Figure 7.1).

A total of 4,032 people participated in the RCTs and 370 participants were in the non-controlled studies. Treatment duration ranged from two to 24 weeks and almost half of the RCTs had a six-week treatment duration. Chinese medicine syndromes were reported in 17 studies, the most common syndrome was Liver *qi* stagnation. Other syndromes included Heart and Spleen deficiency, Liver *qi* stagnation with Spleen deficiency, *qi* stagnation transforming into heat, phlegm stagnation, and melancholy disturbing the mind.

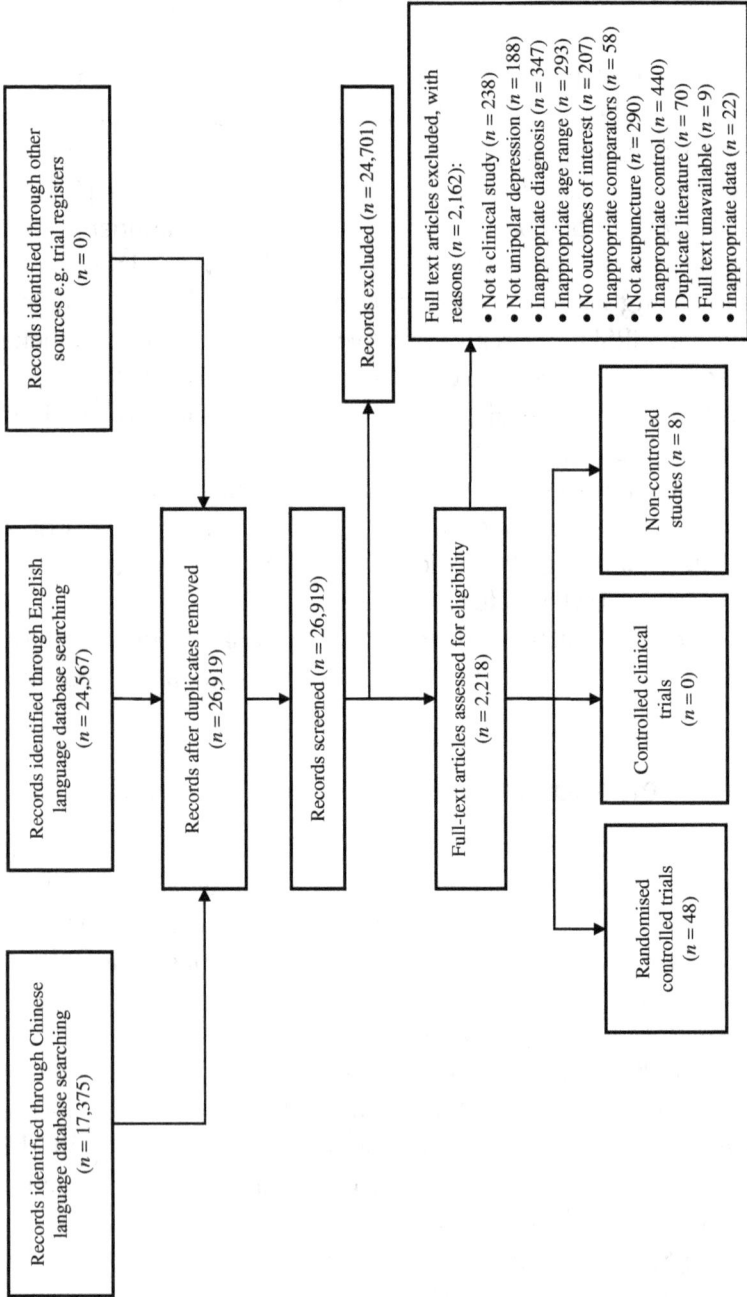

**Figure 7.1.** Flow Chart of Study Selection Process: Acupuncture and Related Therapies

Four different acupuncture therapies were evaluated in the included studies:

- Manual acupuncture (*n* = 33);
- Electroacupuncture (*n* = 15);
- Transcutaneous electrical nerve stimulation (*n* = 2);
- Laser therapy (*n* = 1).

The most frequently reported acupoint across all clinical studies was GV20 *Baihui* 百会 (35 studies). Other commonly used points included: PC6 *Neiguan* 内关 (23 studies), EX-HN3 *Yintang* 印堂 (22 studies), LR3 *Taichong* 太冲 (20 studies), SP6 *Sanyinjiao* 三阴交 (15 studies), and HT7 *Shenmen* 神门 (12 studies).

# Risk of Bias

All 48 RCTs were described as randomised; 30 studies reported adequate details of sequence generation, and two studies used inappropriate methods including alternating or odd and even numbers (A11, A43), and were judged at "high" risk of bias for this domain (Table 7.1). For allocation concealment, only six studies clearly stated the appropriate method of concealment (A4, A13, A20, A25, A27, A28). The remaining studies did not provide sufficient information. Six studies adequately

Table 7.1.  Risk of Bias of Randomised Controlled Trials

| Risk of Bias Domain | Low Risk n (%) | Unclear Risk n (%) | High Risk n (%) |
|---|---|---|---|
| Sequence generation | 30 (62.5) | 16 (33.3) | 2 (4.2) |
| Allocation concealment | 6 (12.5) | 42 (87.5) | 0 (0) |
| Blinding of participants | 6 (12.5) | 2 (4.2) | 40 (83.3) |
| Blinding of personnel* | 3 (6.3) | 2 (4.2) | 43 (89.6) |
| Blinding of outcome assessors | 15 (31.3) | 1 (2.0) | 32 (66.7) |
| Incomplete outcome data | 48 (100) | 0 (0) | 0 (0) |
| Selective outcome reporting | 0 (0) | 48 (100) | 0 (0) |

*Blinding of personnel (acupuncturists) is challenging in manual therapy studies.

described the procedure for blinding of participants using sham acupuncture, sham electroacupuncture or sham laser (A11, A13, A16, A27, A38, A39). Blinding of personnel is difficult in acupuncture studies; however, this was done in three studies that used sham electroacupuncture or laser equipment (A13, A16, A27). Fifteen studies provided descriptions of assessor blinding and was judged as "low" risk of bias (A4, A5, A13, A16, A18, A20, A25–A27, A29–A32, A37, A39). All studies provided detailed information on dropouts and methods of data imputation where appropriate. Therefore, this domain was judged as "low" risk of bias for all studies. No protocol could be located, so all studies were judged as "unclear" risk of bias for selective outcome reporting. Overall, the judgment of the methodological quality of the included studies was limited by inadequate study details.

# Acupuncture

Thirty-nine studies studied the effect of acupuncture for depression; 33 studies were RCTs (A1, A2, A4–A6, A9, A10, A12–A14, A17–A25, A28, A30, A32–A36, A38, A40–A42, A44, A45, A47) and six were non-controlled studies (A49–A52, A55, A56).

## Randomised Controlled Trials of Acupuncture

Twenty-two studies compared acupuncture to antidepressants alone; 10 studies assessed acupuncture as integrative medicine and two studies compared acupuncture to sham/placebo. A total of 2,757 people participated in the studies, treatment duration ranged from four to 24 weeks and the majority of studies (15) had a treatment duration of six weeks. Ten studies reported syndrome differentiation, and the most common syndromes were Liver *qi* stagnation and Heart and Spleen deficiency.

### Acupuncture vs. Antidepressants

### *Hamilton Rating Scale for Depression*

Three versions of the HRSD were used in the included studies; HRSD-17, HRSD-21, and HRSD-24. All studies using a HRSD were grouped together and standard mean difference (SMD) was used for meta-analysis. Different HRSD versions were also subgrouped.

Twenty-one studies (1,656 participants) compared acupuncture with antidepressants. The HRSD score for those who received acupuncture was significantly reduced, compared to antidepressants, indicating reduced depression severity (SMD: −0.23 [−0.46, −0.01], $I^2$ = 79.7%). Subgroup analysis was conducted to explore heterogeneity (Table 7.2). Ten studies (969 participants) used the HRSD-24. Acupuncture was significantly better than antidepressants (mean difference (MD) = −1.38 [−2.68, −0.07, $I^2$ = 84.5%]). The HRSD-17 was also used in 10 studies (607 participants) and there was significant difference between

Table 7.2. Acupuncture vs. Antidepressant: Hamilton Rating Scale for Depression

| Subgroup | No. of Studies (Participants) | MD or SMD [95% CI], $I^2$% | Included Studies |
|---|---|---|---|
| All studies | 21 (1,656) | SMD: −0.23 [−0.46, −0.01]*, $I^2$ = 79.7% | A2, A4–A6, A9, A12, A13, A17, A21, A23, A24, A28, A30, A32, A33, A36, A40, A41, A42, A45, A47 |
| HRSD-17 | 10 (607) | MD: −1.56 [−3.00, −0.11], $I^2$ = 79.8% | A4, A9, A12, A13, A24, A28, A36, A40, A41, A47 |
| HRSD-24 | 10 (969) | MD: −1.38 [−2.68, −0.07], $I^2$ = 84.5% | A2, A5, A6, A17, A21, A23, A32, A33, A42, A45 |
| Low risk of bias: Sequence generation | 13 (1,007) | SMD: −0.13 [−0.46, 0.21], $I^2$ = 84.2% | A2, A4, A13, A17, A21, A23, A24, A28, A30, A32, A33, A40, A47 |
| Treatment duration: ≤6 weeks | 14 (1,173) | SMD: −0.27 [−0.54, 0.00], $I^2$ = 79.7% | A2, A5, A6, A17, A23, A24, A30, A33, A36, A40, A41, A42, A45, A47 |
| Treatment duration: >6 weeks | 7 (483) | SMD: −0.16 [−0.62, 0.30], $I^2$ = 82.6% | A4, A9, A12, A13, A21, A28, A32 |

*(Continued)*

**Table 7.2.** (*Continued*)

| Subgroup | No. of Studies (Participants) | MD or SMD [95% CI], I²% | Included Studies |
|---|---|---|---|
| Verses SSRIs | 20 (1,592) | SMD: –0.25 [–0.49, –0.01]*, I² = 80.5% | A2, A4, A5, A6, A9, A12, A13, A17, A21, A23, A24, A28, A30, A33, A36, A40, A41, A42, A45, A47 |
| Verses fluoxetine | 18 (1,512) | SMD: –0.31 [–0.53, –0.09]*, I² = 76% | A2, A5, A6, A9, A12, A17, A21, A23, A24, A28, A30, A33, A36, A40, A41, A42, A45, A47 |
| Verses escitalopram | 2 (80) | SMD: 0.33 [–1.53, 2.18], I² = 90.3% | A4, A13 |
| Menopause | 7 (631) | SMD: –0.01 [–0.50, 0.48], I² = 87.9% | A5, A6, A12, A13, A24, A33, A47 |
| Postpartum | 2 (112) | SMD: –0.36 [–1.03, 0.31], I² = 68.2% | A2, A41 |

*Statistically significant.

Abbreviations: HRSD, Hamilton Rating Scale for Depression; MD, Mean difference; SMD, standardised mean difference; SSRIs, selective serotonin reuptake inhibitors.

acupuncture and antidepressants (MD: –1.56 [–3.00, –0.11], I² = 79.8%). Heterogeneity was "high" in all subgroups.

Thirteen studies (1,007 participants) had a "low" risk of bias for sequence generation and were subgrouped. However, there was no significant difference between acupuncture and antidepressants (SMD: –0.13 [–0.46, 0.21], I² = 84.2%). Subgroup analyses by treatment duration of less than or equal to six weeks, or greater than six weeks did not reduce heterogeneity nor produce a significant difference between groups.

Twenty studies compared acupuncture to SSRIs (1,592 participants). Meta-analysis showed that acupuncture significantly reduced HRSD scores, compared to SSRIs (SMD: –0.25 [–0.49, –0.01], $I^2$ = 80.5%). Eighteen of these studies (1,512 participants) compared acupuncture to the SSRI fluoxetine and HRSD scores were better after acupuncture (SMD: –0.31 [–0.53, –0.09], $I^2$ = 76%). Another SSRI, escitalopram, was assessed in two studies; no difference was found between acupuncture and escitalopram (SMD: 0.33 [–1.53, 2.18], $I^2$ = 90.3%).

Seven studies assessed depression during menopause (A5, A6, A12, A13, A24, A33, A47) (631 participants). The HRSD score for those who received acupuncture was not significantly better, compared to antidepressants (SMD: –0.01 [–0.50, 0.48], $I^2$ = 87.9%).

Two studies assessed postpartum depression in 112 participants (A2, A41). The HRSD score was not significantly different between the acupuncture and antidepressant groups (SMD –0.36 [–1.03, 0.31], $I^2$ = 68.2%).

## World Health Organization Quality of Life Questionnaire

One study (A18) compared acupuncture to antidepressants in 101 participants. Results showed that acupuncture significantly improved World Health Organization (WHO) quality of life scores compared to antidepressants (MD: 2.7 [0.32, 5.08]).

## Acupuncture Plus Antidepressants vs. Antidepressants

Ten studies (701 participants) compared acupuncture plus antidepressants to antidepressants alone (integrative medicine) (A1, A10, A14, A19, A20, A22, A25, A38, A40, A44).

## Hamilton Rating Scale for Depression

The HRSD scores in the acupuncture groups significantly improved, compared to antidepressants (SMD: –0.84 [–1.17, –0.52], $I^2$ = 70.1%). Subgroup analysis was conducted to explore heterogeneity between studies.

Meta-analysis was possible in six studies that used HRSD-17. The results showed that acupuncture plus antidepressants was significantly better than antidepressants alone (MD: −2.99 [−4.16, −1.82], I² = 39.3%). Four studies (235 participants) (A1, A14, A20, A39), at "low" risk of bias for sequence generation, showed a significant difference between acupuncture plus antidepressants and antidepressant alone (SMD: −0.85 [−1.16, −0.54], I² = 17.3%).

All studies had treatment durations of less than six weeks and it was not possible to conduct subgroup analysis based on treatment duration. All comparator drugs were SSRIs, therefore subgroup analyses was not possible based on drug class. Specific drugs were subgrouped and they all produced a significant difference in HRSD scores when acupuncture was used in combination with the drug, compared to the drug alone, except for sertraline (Table 7.3). There were no depression subgroups such as menopause or postpartum depression. One study

**Table 7.3. Acupuncture Plus Antidepressants vs. Antidepressants: Hamilton Rating Scale for Depression**

| Subgroup | No. of Studies (Participants) | Effect Size (MD or SMD [95% CI], I²%) | Included Studies |
|---|---|---|---|
| All studies | 8 (501) | SMD: −0.84 [−1.17, −0.52]*, I² = 70.1% | A1, A10, A14, A19, A20, A22, A40, A44 |
| HRSD-17 | 6 (301) | MD: −2.99 [−4.16, −1.82]*, I² = 39.3% | A1, A14, A19, A20, A22, A40 |
| Low risk of bias: Sequence generation | 4 (235) | SMD: −0.85 [−1.16, −0.54]*, I² = 17.3% | A1, A14, A20, A40 |
| Verses paroxetine | 3 (193) | SMD: −0.77 [−1.06, −0.47]*, I² = 0.0% | A1, A14, A20 |
| Verses fluoxetine | 3 (242) | SMD: −1.29 [−1.58, −1.01]*, I² = 0.0% | A10, A40, A44 |
| Verses sertraline | 1 (52) | SMD: −0.07 [−0.62, 0.47] | A19 |
| Verses escitalopram | 1 (90) | MD: −0.45 [−0.87, −0.03]* | A22 |

*Statistically significant.

Abbreviations: HRSD, Hamilton Rating Scale for Depression; MD, Mean difference; SMD, standardised mean difference.

(A20) found significant difference between groups at the end of 4 weeks follow-up period (MD = –2.47 [–4.42, –0.5]).

## Montgomery–Asberg Depression Scale

One study compared acupuncture plus fluoxetine, to fluoxetine alone, in 36 participants (A38). Results showed that acupuncture, as integrative medicine, significantly improved Montgomery–Asberg Depression Scale (MADRs) score compared to fluoxetine alone (MD: –8.62 [–9.38, –7.87]).

## Zung Self-rating Depression Scale

One study investigated the effect of acupuncture plus fluoxetine, compared to fluoxetine alone, in 36 participants (A38). Results showed that acupuncture as integrative medicine significantly improved Zung self-rating depression scale (SDS) scores (MD: –9.69 [–10.93, –8.45]).

## Relapse Rate

One study reported on relapse rate at 12 weeks follow-up. Acupuncture significantly reduced depression relapse rate in participants compared to fluoxetine (risk ratio: 0.21 [0.05, 0.90]).

## Controlled Clinical Trials of Acupuncture

No non-randomised CCTs of acupuncture for depression were identified.

## Non-controlled Studies of Acupuncture

Acupuncture therapies were described in six non-controlled clinical studies with a total of 256 participants. One study assessed acupuncture, combined with antidepressants (A50), and the other studies assessed acupuncture alone (A49, A51, A52, A55, A56). Of the three studies that reported CM syndromes, all reported Liver *qi* stagnation, while two reported Liver *qi* stagnation with Spleen deficiency and

Spleen and Heart deficiency (A49, A51, A55). The most commonly used acupuncture points were GV20 *Baihui* 百会 (6 studies), PC6 *Neiguan* 内关 (6 studies), and GV24 *Shenting* 神庭 (4 studies).

## Safety of Acupuncture

Thirteen acupuncture RCTs reported adverse events (AEs) (A1, A2, A5, A12, A13, A20, A21, A23–A25, A34, A35, A48). When compared to placebo, five cases of needle fainting were reported in the acupuncture group. In RCTs that compared acupuncture to antidepressants, no AEs were reported in the acupuncture groups in four studies (A2, A5, A12, A23). The total number of AEs in the acupuncture group was six, and 147 in the antidepressant group. AEs in the acupuncture group included local bruising, needle fainting, dizziness, and tachycardia.

In studies that used acupuncture as integrative medicine, 113 cases of AEs were reported in the integrative medicine group and 122 cases were reported in the antidepressant group in four studies (A1, A20, A25, A48). The most common AEs in the integrative medicine group were tiredness, headache, and gastrointestinal discomfort. The AEs were likely related to concomitant medication, as the antidepressant group reported similar AEs and comparable numbers of AEs.

Three studies included TESS as an AE outcome (A4, A22, A45). Two studies (A4, A45) that compared acupuncture to antidepressants had significantly improved TESS scores (MD: –3.33 [–3.72, –2.95], $I^2$ = 0%); when acupuncture was combined with antidepressants compared to antidepressant alone (A22), TESS scores were also improved (MD: –3.78 [–5.30, –2.26]). However, the studies did not specify the types of AEs.

# Electroacupuncture

A total of 18 studies used electroacupuncture; 16 were RCTs (A3, A7, A8, A13, A15, A16, A18, A20, A25, A26, A29, A31, A37, A39, A43, A46) and two were non-controlled studies (A53, A54).

## Randomised Controlled Trials of Electroacupuncture

Sixteen studies used electroacupuncture as intervention. A total of 1,476 people participated in the studies. Three studies had a treatment duration of four weeks or less, 10 studies had a treatment duration of six weeks, two studies had a treatment of eight weeks and one study had a treatment period of 24 weeks. Four studies reported CM syndrome differentiation, the most common syndrome was Liver *qi* stagnation. Other syndromes included Heart and Spleen deficiency, Liver *qi* stagnation with Spleen deficiency, *qi* stagnation transforming into heat, phlegm stagnation, and melancholy disturbing the mind.

## Electroacupuncture vs. Sham Electroacupuncture

Three studies (A16, A29, A39) compared electroacupuncture to sham electroacupuncture (201 participants).

### *Hamilton Rating Scale for Depression*

Meta-analysis showed that electroacupuncture significantly improved HRSD scores (SMD: −0.34 [−0.65, −0.04], $I^2 = 0\%$).

### *Zung Self-rating Depression Scale*

One study (A16) assessed SDS scores in 63 participants. Electroacupuncture was superior to sham electroacupuncture after six weeks of treatment (MD: −6.98 [−12.60, −1.37]).

## Electroacupuncture vs. Antidepressants

Seven studies (718 participants) compared electroacupuncture to antidepressants.

### *Hamilton Rating Scale for Depression*

HRSD scores were not significantly different when electroacupuncture was compared to antidepressants alone (SMD: −0.28, [−0.66,

0.10], $I^2$ = 78.8%). The HRSD-24 was used in four studies (338 participants) and meta-analysis showed a significant difference between electroacupuncture and antidepressants (MD: −2.55 [−3.43, −1.66], $I^2$ = 18.8%). Two studies (285 participants) used HRSD-17 and meta-analysis results did not show a significant difference between groups (MD: 0.89 [−0.27, 2.04], $I^2$ = 0%) (Table 7.4).

Four studies had a low risk of bias for sequence generation and did not show a significant difference between electro-acupuncture and antidepressants (Table 7.4). Six studies had a treatment duration of less than, or equal to, six weeks and did not show a significant difference of HRSD scores between electroacupuncture and antidepressants. All studies used SSRIs as a comparator and subgroup analysis was not possible based on drug class.

Table 7.4. Electroacupuncture vs. Antidepressants: Hamilton Rating Scale for Depression

| Subgroup | No. of Studies (Participants) | Effect Size (MD or SMD [95% CI], $I^2$%) | Included Studies |
|---|---|---|---|
| All studies | 7 (718) | SMD: −0.28 [−0.66, 0.10], $I^2$ = 78.8% | A3, A13, A15, A16, A26, A29, A46 |
| HRSD-24 | 4 (338) | MD: −2.55 [−3.43, −1.66], $I^2$ = 18.8% | A3, A15, A29, A46 |
| HRSD-17 | 2 (285) | MD: 0.89 [−0.27, 2.04], $I^2$ = 0% | A13, A26 |
| Low risk of bias: Sequence generation | 4 (403) | SMD: −0.18 [−0.67, 0.31], $I^2$ = 76.8% | A3, A13, A26, A46 |
| Treatment duration: ≤6 weeks | 6 (628) | SMD: −0.36 [−0.76, 0.05], $I^2$ = 79.8% | A3, A15, A16, A26, A29, A46 |
| Menopause | 1 (60) | MD: 0.58 [−1.01, 2.17]) | A13 |

*Statistically significant.

Abbreviations: HRSD, Hamilton Rating Scale for Depression; MD, Mean difference; SMD, standardised mean difference.

In menopausal women (A13), the mean HRSD-17 score for those who received electroacupuncture was not significantly better than antidepressants (MD: 0.58 [–1.01, 2.17]). One study had a follow-up of 12 weeks (A13). There was no significant difference in HRSD-17 score between groups (MD: –1.74 [–3.51, 0.03]).

## Zung Self-rating Depression Scale

Three studies assessed the SDS and compared electroacupuncture to SSRIs after six weeks treatment (A16, A26, A46). Those who received electroacupuncture did not have improved SDS scores compared to antidepressants (MD: –3.08 [–16.99, 10.84], $I^2$ = 98.5%).

## World Health Organization Quality of Life Questionnaire

One study (A20) assessed the WHO quality of life questionnaire. Compared to antidepressants, electroacupuncture was not superior (MD: 2 [–0.23, 4.23]).

## Electroacupuncture Plus Antidepressants vs. Antidepressants

Six studies (477 participants) compared electroacupuncture plus anti-depressant to antidepressants alone (A7, A8, A20, A26, A31, A43).

## Hamilton Rating Scale for Depression

The HRSD score for those who received acupuncture significantly improved, compared to antidepressants alone in seven studies (SMD: –0.52 [–0.88, –0.17], $I^2$ = 69.6%). The HRSD-17 was used in five studies (382 participants) and was grouped for meta-analysis (A8, A20, A26, A31, A43). Results showed significant differences between electroacupuncture plus antidepressants, compared to antidepressants alone (MD: –2.28 [–4.06, –0.50], $I^2$ = 72.8%). At the end of follow-up in two studies (A20, A31), significant differences were found between the treatment groups (MD –2.86 [4.29, –1.44], $I^2$ = 0%).

### *Zung Self-rating Depression Scale*

Two studies (A8, A26), with 189 participants, assessed SDS. Electroacupuncture plus antidepressants did not improve the SDS scores more than antidepressants alone (MD: −2.01 [−10.42, 6.40], $I^2$ = 85.3%).

### Electroacupuncture vs. Psychotherapy

One study (A37), with 60 participants, compared electroacupuncture to cognitive behavioural therapy. The HRSD-17 scores were not different between groups (MD: −0.44 [−2.06, 1.18]).

### Electroacupuncture Plus Psychotherapy vs. Psychotherapy

One study (A37), with 60 participants, compared electroacupuncture plus cognitive behavioural therapy to cognitive behavioural therapy alone.The HRSD-17 scores improved significantly (MD: −2.30 [−3.89, −0.71]).

### Controlled Clinical Trials of Electroacupuncture

No non-randomised CCT of acupuncture for depression were included in the analysis.

### Non-controlled Studies of Electroacupuncture

Electroacupuncture therapies were assessed in two non-controlled clinical studies with a total of 114 participants (A53, A54). One study reported electroacupuncture combined with cognitive behavioural therapy (A53) and one study assessed electroacupuncture alone (A54). Chinese medicine syndromes were not reported. The acupoint GV20 *Baihui* 百会 was used in both studies.

### Safety of Electroacupuncture

Seven electroacupuncture RCTs reported on AEs (A3, A12, A20, A25, A26, A39, A43). One study reported more AEs in the sham electroacupuncture group compared to the electroacupuncture group (A39). In RCTs that compared electroacupuncture to antidepressants, one study did not report any AEs in the acupuncture group (A3). Two RCTs reported headache (2 cases), local hematoma (2), and dizziness (1) (A13, A16). One study reported one AE in the electroacupuncture group but did not provide any information (A26).

When electroacupuncture was studied as integrative medicine, AEs were mentioned in four RCTs (A20, A25, A26, A39). However, in some studies the information on the type or number of each AE was incomplete (A20, A26). Tiredness, sleep disturbance and headache were the most common AEs reported in the integrative medicine group. The antidepressant groups reported similar AEs and comparable numbers.

Two studies assessed TESS scores when electroacupuncture plus antidepressants were compared to antidepressants alone, in 137 participants (A7, A43). The results showed that electroacupuncture as integrative medicine did not improve TESS scores, compared to antidepressants alone (MD: −2.74 [−8.52, 3.03], $I^2$ = 99.4%). Two studies assessed SERS scores in 190 participants (A1, A20). Results showed that electroacupuncture as integrative medicine did not improve SERS scores, compared to antidepressants alone (MD: −2.09 [−4.38, 0.21], $I^2$ = 71.4%).

# Acupuncture-related Therapies

## Transcutaneous Electrical Nerve Stimulation

One RCT combined stimulation on PC6 *Neiguan* 内关 plus sertraline to sertraline alone in 60 participants (A48). Acupoint stimulation plus antidepressants did not improve the HRSD-24 scores more than antidepressants alone (MD: 10.03 [8.63, 11.43]). The study did not report on AEs.

One RCT compared ear-TENS with sham ear-TENS (A11). Ear-TENS did not improve the HRSD-17 scores in 22 participants after 40 days of treatment (MD: −2.3 [−8.06, 3.46]). However, ear-TENS significantly improved Beck Depression Inventory Scores (MD: −11.8 [−21.85, −1.75]). The study did not report on AEs.

### Laser Therapy

One RCT assessed 47 participants and compared laser acupuncture therapy to placebo laser therapy (A27). Laser acupuncture points included: LR14 *Qimen* 期门, CV14 *Juque* 巨阙, LR8 *Ququan* 曲泉, HT7 *Shenmen* 神门, and KI3 *Taixi* 太溪. Laser improved the HRSD-17 scores, compared to placebo, after eight weeks treatment (MD: –4.86 [–8.11, –1.61]). The study reported AEs but did not specify the number of events in each group. AEs in the laser acupuncture group were minimal, including transient fatigue, and in the placebo group events included aches, transient fatigue, and vagueness.

# Frequently Reported Acupuncture Points in Meta-analyses Showing Favourable Effect

Based on outcome category, the most frequently reported acupuncture points in meta-analyses showing favourable effect were: GV20 *Baihui* 百会 (30 studies), EX-HN3 *Yintang* 印堂 (20 studies), PC6 *Neiguan* 内关 (16 studies), LR3 *Taichong* 太冲 (14 studies), SP6 *Sanyinjiao* 三阴交 (14 studies), BL18 *Ganshu* 肝俞 (13 studies), HT7 *Shenmen* 神门 (11 studies), and GV24 *Shenting* 神庭 (7 studies).

# Assessment Using GRADE

An assessment of the quality of the evidence from RCTs was made using GRADE. Interventions, comparators and outcomes to be included were selected based on a consensus process, described in Chapter 4. Comparisons were: Acupuncture versus antidepressants and acupuncture plus antidepressants versus antidepressants alone. Note that acupuncture studies and electroacupuncture studies were merged in the GRADE analysis.

Evidence for acupuncture versus antidepressants was "low" to "very low" quality (Table 7.5). The results showed that acupuncture-may reduce depression severity.

Evidence for acupuncture plus antidepressants versus antidepressants alone was "low" to "very low" quality (Table 7.6). The results showed that acupuncture may reduce depression severity.

**Table 7.5.  GRADE: Acupuncture vs. Antidepressants**

| Outcomes | No. of Participants (Studies) | Certainty of the Evidence (GRADE) | Anticipated Absolute Effects | |
|---|---|---|---|---|
| | | | Risk with Antidepressants | Risk Difference with Acupuncture |
| Hamilton Rating Scale for Depression | 2,039 (27 RCTs) | ⊕⊕◯◯ LOW[1,2] | — | SMD **0.28 SD lower** (0.46 lower to 0.09 lower) |
| Treatment duration: Mean 6.8 weeks | | | | |
| Self-rating Depression Scale | 250 (3 RCTs) | ⊕◯◯◯ VERY LOW[1,2,3] | The mean Self-rating Depression Scale was **48.75 points** | MD **4.39 points lower** (15.74 lower to 6.95 higher) |
| Scale from: 20 to 80 | | | | |
| Treatment duration: Mean 6 weeks | | | | |
| Adverse events | 747 (9 RCTs) | | Five RCTs reported no adverse events in the acupuncture group. Nine studies reported a total of seven adverse events, including local bruising (2), needle fainting (2), dizziness (1) headache (1) and tachycardia (1). The antidepressant groups reported 174 adverse events including dry mouth (20), tiredness (17), headache (17), dizziness (14), nausea (12), and insomnia (10). Two studies (A4, A46) significantly improved TESS scores (MD: −3.33 [−3.72, −2.95], I² = 0%). | |

*The risk in the intervention group (and its 95% confidence interval) is based on the assumed risk in the comparison group and the relative effect of the intervention (and its 95% CI).

Abbreviations: CI, confidence interval; GRADE, Grading of Recommendations Assessment, Development and Evaluation; MD, mean difference; RCTs, randomised controlled trials; SMD, standardised mean difference; TESS, Treatment Emergent Symptom Scale.

*Notes:*

1. Unclear sequence generation and allocation concealment. Lack of blinding of participants and personnel;
2. Considerable statistical heterogeneity;
3. Wide confidence interval and small sample size.

*Study References*

Hamilton Rating Scale for Depression (HRSD): A2–A6, A9, A12, A13, A15–A17, A21, A23, A24, A26, A28–A30, A32, A33, A36, A40–A42, A45–A47;
Self-rating Depression Scale (SDS): A16, A26, A46;
Adverse events: A2, A3, A5, A12, A13, A21, A23, A24, A26.

**Table 7.6. GRADE: Acupuncture Plus Antidepressants vs. Antidepressants**

| Outcomes | No. of Participants (Studies) | Certainty of the Evidence (GRADE) | Anticipated Absolute Effects | |
|---|---|---|---|---|
| | | | Risk with Antidepressants | Risk Difference with Acupuncture + Antidepressants |
| **Hamilton Rating Scale for Depression** Treatment duration: Mean 6.8 weeks | 463 (13 RCTs) | ⊕⊕○○ LOW[1,2] | — | SMD **0.69 SD lower** (0.96 lower to 0.42 lower) |
| **Self-rating Depression Scale** Scale from: 20 to 80 Treatment duration: 8 weeks | 110 (3 RCTs) | ⊕○○○ VERY LOW[1,3] | The mean Self-rating Depression Scale was 44.07 points | MD **3.5 points lower** (14.36 lower to 7.36 higher) |
| **Adverse events** | 678 (6 RCTs) | | The integrative group had a total of 192 adverse events including tiredness (27), sleep disturbance (21), gastrointestinal discomfort (7), and headache (7). The antidepressant groups reported 141 adverse events including tiredness (28), sleep disturbance (28), headache (13), and dry mouth (7). Three studies (A7, A22, A44) assessed TESS scores but there was no significant differences between groups (MD: −3.08 [−7.41, 1.25], $I^2$ = 98.8%). Three studies (A1, A20, A26) had significantly improved SERS scores (MD: −2.61 [−4.43, −0.78], $I^2$ = 80.9%). | |

*The risk in the intervention group (and its 95% confidence interval) is based on the assumed risk in the comparison group and the relative effect of the intervention (and its 95% CI).

Abbreviations: CI, confidence interval; GRADE, Grading of Recommendations Assessment, Development and Evaluation; MD, mean difference; RCTs, randomised controlled trials; SERS, Side-Effect Rating Scale; SMD, standardised mean difference; TESS, Treatment Emergent Symptom Scale.

Notes:

1. Unclear sequence generation and allocation concealment. Lack of blinding of participants and personnel;
2. Considerable statistical heterogeneity;
3. Wide confidence interval and small sample size.

Study References

Hamilton Rating Scale for Depression (HRSD): A1, A7, A8, A10, A14, A19, A20, A22, A26, A31, A40, A43, A44;
Self-rating Depression Scale (SDS): A8, A26, A38;
Adverse events: A1, A20, A25, A26, A43, A44.

# Summary of Acupuncture and Related Therapies

Acupuncture for the management of depression has been evaluated in RCTs and non-controlled studies. Manual acupuncture and electroacupuncture were the two main types of acupuncture therapies used in clinical trials. Many studies reported on depression severity scales, including HRSD, SDS, and MADRS. Some studies reported health-related quality of life outcomes. Meta-analyses was possible for various comparisons and outcomes.

Meta-analyses showed that the effectiveness of acupuncture may be similar to antidepressants, in terms of depression symptom severity measured with the HRSD, SDS, and MADRS. These findings were seen when manual acupuncture or electroacupuncture was used alone, or as integrative medicine. Findings from a single study that assessed quality of life did not show benefit of acupuncture or electroacupuncture greater than control. Therefore, the effect on quality of life in people with depression is unknown.

Meta-analyses results showed statistical heterogeneity and subgroup analysis did not explain the reason for heterogeneity. This suggests that there was considerable variability in the studies. This may be expected since the included studies used different combinations of acupuncture points, different methods of point stimulation, and there were a number of different comparators. Further to this, differences exist in the participant groups in relation to duration and severity of depression, as well as in the duration and frequency of treatment. All these factors limit confidence in the results and contributed to the downgrading of the evidence in GRADE.

Liver *qi* stagnation and Heart and Spleen deficiency were the most commonly reported syndromes in clinical studies. Commonly used acupuncture points in clinical trials with a favourable effect included: GV20 *Baihui* 百会, HT7 *Shenmen* 神门, PC6 *Neiguan* 内关, LR3 *Taichong* 太冲, SP6 *Sanyinjiao* 三阴交, and BL18 *Ganshu* 肝俞.

In studies that reported AEs, acupuncture therapies appear to be well-tolerated by people with depression. The number of AEs was low when acupuncture or electroacupuncture was assessed alone. In the case of acupuncture therapies combined with antidepressants, the number of AEs increased dramatically. Common AEs were dry mouth, gastrointestinal discomfort, tiredness, and sleep disturbance. These AEs were not seen in those who received acupuncture alone, suggesting they may be caused by antidepressants.

# References

1. Smith CA, Hay PP and MacPherson H. (2010) Acupuncture for depression. *Cochrane Database Syst Rev* **20**(1): CD004046.
2. Stub T, Alræk T and Liu J. (2011) Acupuncture treatment for depression — A systematic review and meta-analysis. *Eur J Integr Med* **3**(4): e259–e270.
3. Shen H, Zhang J, Yang J and Yang N. (2014) 针刺治疗抑郁症随机对照研究的系统评价. *Journal of New Chinese Medicine* **1**(46).
4. Zhang ZJ, Chen HY, Yip KC, *et al.* (2010) The effectiveness and safety of acupuncture therapy in depressive disorders: systematic review and meta-analysis. *J Affect Disord* **124**(1–2): 9–21.
5. Chan YY, Lo WY, Yang SN, *et al.* (2015) The benefit of combined acupuncture and antidepressant medication for depression: A systematic review and meta-analysis. *J Affect Disord* **176**: 106–117.
6. Zhang Y, Qu SS, Zhang JP, *et al.* (2016) Rapid Onset of the Effects of Combined Selective Serotonin Reuptake Inhibitors and Electroacupuncture on Primary Depression: a Meta-Analysis. *J Altern Complement Med* **22**(1): 1–8.

**References for Included Acupuncture Therapies: Clinical Studies**

| Study No. | References |
| --- | --- |
| A1 | 陈海东, 杨秀岩, 马学红, 谢占国, 陈万里, 图娅. 针刺联合盐酸帕罗西汀片治疗轻中度抑郁症临床研究. 中国中医药信息杂志, 2014, **21**(08): 35–38. |
| A2 | 陈杰, 张捷, 裴音. 针刺治疗产后抑郁症的疗效评价. 中国中医药信息杂志, 2010, **17**(07): 77–78. |
| A3 | 陈秀玲, 徐凯, 罗仁瀚, 林妙君. 电针四神聪穴治疗抑郁症疗效观察. 上海针灸杂志, 2012, **31**(01): 26–28. |
| A4 | 陈小艳. 针灸对抑郁症患者情绪相关脑区功能的影响. 成都中医药大学, 2015. |
| A5 | 迟慧, 邹伟. 益肾调肝针刺法治疗围绝经期抑郁症30例. 针灸临床杂志, 2011, **27**(07): 4–7. |

**(*Continued*)**

| Study No. | References |
| --- | --- |
| A6 | 丁丽, 刘波. 补肾调肝健脾宁心针法治疗围绝经期抑郁症的临床观察. 中华中医药学刊, 2007, **25**(05):1066–1067. |
| A7 | Duan DM, Tu Y, Chen LP, *et al.* (2009) Efficacy evaluation for depression with somatic symptoms treated by electroacupuncture combined with Fluoxetine. *J Tradit Chin Med* **29**(3): 167–173. |
| A8 | 冯骥. 电针靳三针结合药物文拉法辛治疗抑郁症的临床疗效观察. 黑龙江中医药大学, 2015. |
| A9 | 高红. 针灸解郁方治疗抑郁症疗效分析. 中国误诊学杂志, 2008, **8**(34): 8348–8349. |
| A10 | 高鹏, 吴龙海. 针灸疗法联合氟西汀治疗抑郁障碍的临床疗效观察. 中国医药指南, 2016, **14**(04): 29. |
| A11 | Hein E, Nowak M, Kiess O, *et al.* (2013) Auricular transcutaneous electrical nerve stimulation in depressed patients: a randomized controlled pilot study. *J Neural Transm (Vienna)* **120**(5): 821–827. |
| A12 | 李海波. 针刺治疗肾虚肝郁型围绝经期抑郁症的临床观察. 黑龙江中医药大学, 2015. |
| A13 | 李昭凤. 电针治疗围绝经期轻中度抑郁障碍的临床研究. 广州中医药大学, 2015. |
| A14 | 林月青. 浅针配合盐酸氟西汀治疗肝气郁结型抑郁症的临床研究. 福建中医药大学, 2014. |
| A15 | 刘述霞, 王秀花, 刘秀丽, 张向花, 张蕾. 电针治疗抑郁症118例. 中医研究, 2010, **23**(09): 76–77. |
| A16 | 罗和春, Ureil Halbriech, 沈渔邨, 孟凡强, 赵学英, 梁炜, 谭春香, 韩毳, 周东丰, 刘平. 电针与氟西汀治疗抑郁症疗效的对照研究. 中华精神科杂志, 2003, **36**(04): 26–30. |
| A17 | 罗仁瀚, 徐凯, 黄云声. 针刺治疗抑郁症临床观察. 上海针灸杂志, 2009, **28**(02): 69–71. |
| A18 | Ma S, Qu S, Huang Y, *et al.* (2012) Improvement in quality of life in depressed patients following verum acupuncture or electroacupuncture plus paroxetine: A randomized controlled study of 157 cases. *Neural Regen Res* **7**(27): 2123–2129. |
| A19 | 马霞. 针刺合并舍曲林治疗抑郁症疗效观察. 四川中医, 2012, **30**(08): 140–141. |
| A20 | 马学红. 针刺抗抑郁的临床研究. 北京中医药大学, 2011. |

(*Continued*)

**(Continued)**

| Study No. | References |
|---|---|
| A21 | 苗萌萌, 吴俊梅. "疏肝健脾、通督调心" 针法治疗肝气郁结型抑郁障碍疗效观察. 中医药临床杂志, 2015, **27**(08): 1115–1117. |
| A22 | 潘玉印. 穴位针刺联合氢溴酸西酞普兰治疗复发性抑郁症的对照研究. 精神医学杂志, 2014, **27**(01): 24–26. |
| A23 | 裴音, 张捷, 陈杰, 钱洁. 针刺王氏五脏俞治疗抑郁症临床观察. 中国中医药信息杂志, 2006, **13**(06): 62–63. |
| A24 | 钱洁, 张捷, 裴音, 陈杰. 王氏五脏俞加膈俞治疗更年期抑郁症的临床观察. 北京中医, 2007, **26**(08): 491–492. |
| A25 | Qu SS, Huang Y, Zhang ZJ, *et al.* (2013) A 6-week randomized controlled trial with 4-week follow-up of acupuncture combined with paroxetine in patients with major depressive disorder. *J Psychiatr Res* **47**(6): 726–732. |
| A26 | 曲姗姗. 电针印堂、百会治疗轻中度原发性抑郁症的临床观察及 Rs-fMRI 研究. 南方医科大学, 2015. |
| A27 | Quah-Smith I, Smith C, Crawford JD, *et al.* (2013) Laser acupuncture for depression: a randomised double blind controlled trial using low intensity laser intervention. *J Affect Disord* **148**(2–3): 179–187. |
| A28 | 石彧, 王志祥, 周哲屹, 卢昌均. 泻肝补肺针法治疗太阴人抑郁症的临床研究. 南京中医药大学学报, 2015, **31**(02): 118–121. |
| A29 | Song Y, Zhou D, Fan J, *et al.* (2007) Effects of electroacupuncture and fluoxetine on the density of GTP-binding-proteins in platelet membrane in patients with major depressive disorder. *J Affect Disord* **98**(3): 253–257. |
| A30 | 宋书昌, 卢智, 陈华, 王利春, 张全围. 形神合治针法治疗抑郁症 40 例疗效观察. 针灸临床杂志 2013, **29**(09): 27–29. |
| A31 | 汪崇琦. 电针结合帕罗西汀治疗抑郁症的临床观察. 南方医科大学, 2010. |
| A32 | 王群松, 季向东, 朱文娴, 于海燕. 针刺治疗对阴虚火旺型抑郁症的血清 BDNF 影响. 首都医科大学学报, 2016, **37**(02): 176–180. |
| A33 | 邢凯. 醒神解郁针法治疗女性更年期抑郁症120例临床观察. 中国妇幼保健, 2011, **26**(34): 5373–5375. |
| A34 | 徐峰. 逍遥散配合针灸治疗产后抑郁症的临床研究. 世界中西医结合杂志, 2013, **8**(09): 896–899. |
| A35 | 许芳, 唐启盛, 李小黎. 益肾调气法治疗产后抑郁症的随机对照临床研究. 北京中医药, 2013, **32**(03): 200–203. |
| A36 | 徐凤鸣, 王奇, 刘晓磊. 针刺治疗抑郁症的临床观察. 针灸临床杂志, 2009, **25**(09): 27–28. |

**(*Continued*)**

| Study No. | References |
|---|---|
| A37 | 杨学琴, 张文悦, 马文昊, 郭天蔚, 秦丽娜, 杨昕婧, 王思涵, 图娅. 电针联合认知行为疗法早期干预轻度抑郁状态30例疗效观察. 中医杂志, 2012, **53**(11): 936–938+968. |
| A38 | 叶郭锡. 腹针联合药物对抑郁症脑功能连接的磁共振研究. 广州中医药大学, 2015. |
| A39 | Yeung WF, Chung KF, Tso KC, *et al.* (2011) Electroacupuncture for residual insomnia associated with major depressive disorder: a randomized controlled trial. *Sleep* **34**(6): 807–815. |
| A40 | 易洋, 徐放明, 谢洪武, 宋云娥, 吕发金, 谢鹏, 杨德兰, 林云, 冯伟, 胡皓, 孙娟. 从针刺太冲穴治疗抑郁症探讨肝经与额叶联系的静息态功能磁共振研究. 中国中西医结合杂志, 2011, **31**(08): 1044–1050. |
| A41 | 于树静, 李雪青, 冯小明, 曹文芳. 针刺十三鬼穴对产后抑郁患者疗效及生活质量的影响. 四川中医, 2015, **33**(03): 163–165. |
| A42 | 余永森. 针刺捻转泻法为主治疗肝气郁结型抑郁症的临床疗效观察. 广州中医药大学, 2012. |
| A43 | Zhang GJ, Shi ZY, Liu S, *et al.* (2007) Clinical observation on treatment of depression by electro-acupuncture combined with Paroxetine. *Chin J Integr Med* **13**(3): 228–230. |
| A44 | 郑艳辉, 侯乐. 醒脑开窍针法联合氟西汀治疗抑郁症的临床疗效观察. 现代诊断与治疗, 2016, **27**(02): 220–222. |
| A45 | 周金平. 针灸治疗抑郁症的临床疗效及安全性评价. 中国医刊, 2013, **48**(02): 90–91. |
| A46 | 周磊. 电项针治疗抑郁症临床研究. 黑龙江中医药大学, 2011. |
| A47 | 周胜红. 针刺治疗女性更年期抑郁症60例. 中国组织工程研究与临床康复, 2007, **17**(39): 7817–7819. |
| A48 | 朱越琪, 郭鸿, 兰建华. 舍曲林联合穴位刺激调控法治疗抑郁症的效果及安全性. 中国医药导报, 2014, **11**(14): 63–65. |
| A49 | 曹铁军, 黄芳, 李霞, 王健. 从奇经论治抑郁症的临床观察. 中华中医药学刊, 2007, (07): 1401–1402. |
| A50 | Guo JQ, Zhou JC, Huang Y, *et al.* (2009) A clinical study on treating primary depression by the combination of acupuncture and paroxetine. *International Journal of Clinical Acupuncture* **18**(4): 229–232. |
| A51 | 黄芳. 从奇经论治抑郁症临床观察. 辽宁中医学院, 2005. |

(*Continued*)

(***Continued***)

| Study No. | References |
|---|---|
| A52 | 马莉, 程为平, 梅晨健, 张洋, 肖飞, 李崖雪. 加强扬刺百会穴对抑郁症患者体内单胺类神经递质代谢影响的研究. 中西医结合心脑血管病杂志, 2012, **10**(05): 562–563. |
| A53 | 张韧, 赵军, 倪国忠, 杨欣鹏. 赵军教授调神解郁针法治疗肝气郁结型青年抑郁症的疗效观察. 中医临床研究, 2014, **6**(13): 37–38. |
| A54 | 张小兰, 姜艳, 殷凤凤. 针刺治疗抑郁症35例. 吉林中医药, 2008, **28**(10): 753. |
| A55 | 黄芳, 曹铁军, 曹锐, 李宝岩. 电针内关、建里治疗抑郁症的临床研究. 北京中医药大学学报(中医临床版), 2008, **15**(02): 25–27. |
| A56 | 沈莉, 颜红. 电针配合认知疗法治疗抑郁症68例疗效观察. 新中医, 2008, **40**(01): 66–68. |

# 8

# Clinical Evidence for Other Chinese Medicine Therapies

## OVERVIEW

Other Chinese medicine therapies for depression include *tuina* 推拿, cupping, *taichi* 太极, and diet therapy. However, there was an overall lack of evidence supporting the use of other Chinese medicine therapies for depression. Only two clinical trials were identified for inclusion in this chapter. They assessed cupping and *tuina* 推拿 for depression.

## Introduction

In addition to Chinese herbal medicine and acupuncture therapies, Chinese medicine (CM) includes a range of other CM therapies to treat disease and maintain health. These include cupping therapy, which involves the application of suction by placing a vaccumised cup onto the body and moving it along the meridian or disease area; *tuina* 推拿, and Chinese massage therapy.

## Previous Systematic Reviews

No systematic reviews were identified in either English or Chinese literature.

## Identification of Clinical Studies

Based on the eligibility criteria, two randomised controlled trials (RCTs) were included (O1-O2, Figure 8.1). Evidence from the RCTs

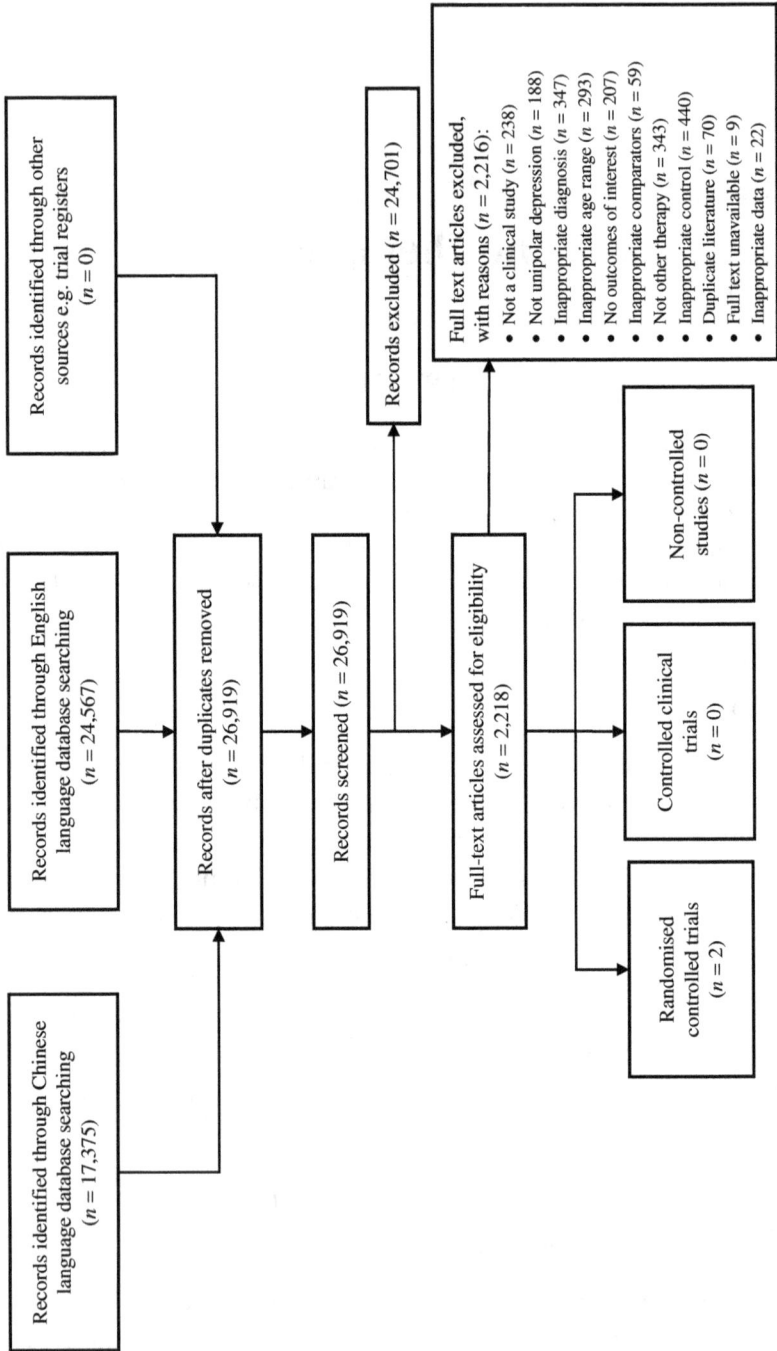

**Figure 8.1.** Flow Chart of Study Selection Process: Other Chinese Medicine Therapies

was evaluated to establish the efficacy and safety of other therapies for depression. Three hundred and fifty-six participants were included in the RCTs. Both studies were conducted in China, with treatment duration of equal to, or less than six weeks. One study compared *tuina* 推拿 to fluoxetine whilst the other study compared mobile cupping plus fluoxetine to fluoxetine alone. The studies did not report CM syndromes.

## Cupping Therapy

One RCT (O2) compared mobile cupping as integrative medicine with fluoxetine alone (116 participants). Mobile cupping was performed along the Governor Vessel and Bladder meridians on the back. The Hamilton Depression Rating Scale (HRSD)-24 scores showed significant differences between the two groups after six weeks of treatment (mean difference (MD): −13.94 [−15.39, −12.49]). Adverse events were reported in both intervention groups and were not significantly different between groups. Adverse events included insomnia, dry mouth, dizziness, palpitations, nausea and vomiting, diarrhoea, and loss of appetite.

## Tuina

One RCT (O1) compared *tuina* 推拿 to fluoxetine (240 participants). *Tuina* 推拿 was performed on acupoints including: GV20 *Baihui* 百会, GV16 *Fengfu* 风府, GB20 *Fengchi* 风池, PC8 *Laogong* 劳工, PC7 *Daling* 大陵, LR3 *Taichong* 太冲, and GB34 *Yanglingquan* 阳陵泉. The HRSD-24 scores showed significant differences between the two groups after six weeks of treatments (MD: −3.52 [−4.86, −2.18]). The study did not report on adverse events.

# Summary of Other Chinese Medicine

The number of studies for depression using other CM therapies is very small despite the extensive search of the literature. This suggests that Chinese herbal medicine and acupuncture are the more frequently used treatment methods for depression. Meta-analysis was not possible for the identified studies as the methods of intervention were different. Both studies found beneficial effects of CM therapies.

**References for Included Other Chinese Medicine Therapies: Clinical Studies**

| Study No. | References |
|-----------|------------|
| O1 | 邢凯, 艾民. 养心安神疏肝推拿法治疗抑郁症120例临床观察. 医学信息, 2013, 26(30): 82. |
| O2 | 张捷, 裴音, 陈杰, 等. 中西医结合治疗抑郁症临床观察. 中国中医药信息杂志, 2005, 12(10): 63–64. |

# 9

# Clinical Evidence for Combination Therapies

**OVERVIEW**

Chinese medicine clinical practice often uses two or more types of therapies together, such as Chinese herbal medicine plus acupuncture. This chapter includes clinical studies that use a combination treatment therapies for depression. Acupuncture was combined with several therapies including Chinese herbal medicine, *tuina* 推拿, and cupping in the included studies and results show benefit for some combinations.

## Introduction

Combination Chinese medicine (CM) therapies are defined as two or more CM interventions from different categories administered together, for example Chinese herbal medicine (CHM) plus acupuncture. This approach is common in clinical practice.

### Randomised Controlled Trials of Combination Therapies

Twelve studies were identified as randomized controlled trials (RCTs) of combination therapies (C1–C12, Figure 9.1). A total of 1,052 participants were included in the studies. The most common syndrome described in the studies was Liver *qi* stagnation. Therapies included:

- Acupuncture plus CHM (7 studies);
- Acupuncture plus *tuina* 推拿 (1 study);
- Acupuncture plus moxibustion (1 study);

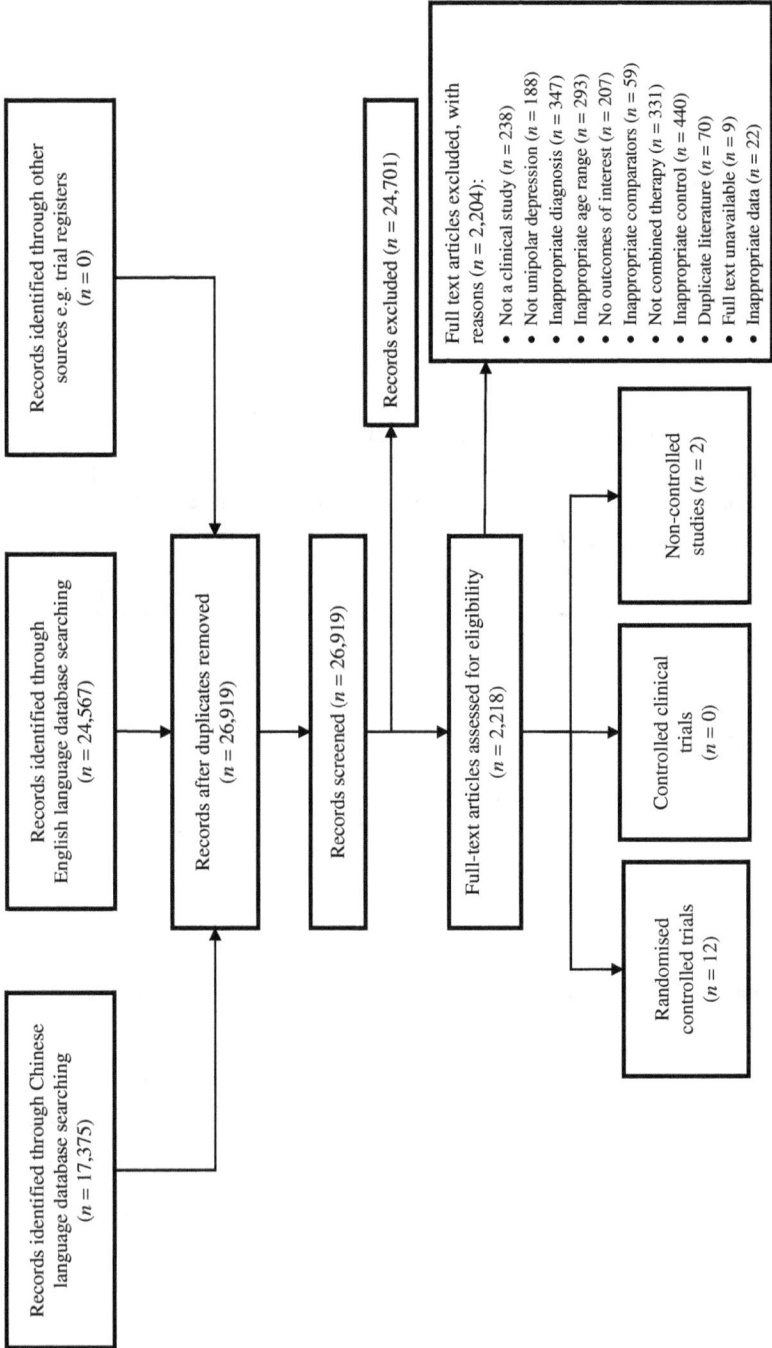

**Figure 9.1.** Flow Chart of Study Selection Process: Combination Therapies

- Acupuncture plus moxibustion plus five element music therapy (1 study);
- Acupuncture plus mobile cupping plus psychotherapy (1 study);
- *Qigong* 气功 plus *taichi* 太极 plus *tuina* 推拿 plus antidepressants (1 study).

# Risk of Bias

Six studies used either computer software or a random number table for sequence generation and were assessed as "low" risk of bias (C1, C3, C4, C6, C7, C11). None of the studies described methods of allocation concealment and were assessed at "unclear" risk. One study mentioned "single blinding" but did not clarify what this meant, therefore was judged at "unclear" risk for blinding of participants, personnel and assessors (C3). The remaining studies were judged as "high" risk for blinding due to the nature of the interventions and comparators. Where applicable, reasons for dropout were reported and dropout numbers were balanced between groups. Therefore, all studies were assessed as "low" risk of bias for incomplete outcome data. No protocols were identified for the included studies and all studies were assessed as "unclear" risk of bias for selective reporting (Table 9.1).

Table 9.1. Risk of Bias of Randomised Controlled Trials: Combination Therapies

| Risk of Bias Domain | Low Risk n (%) | Unclear Risk n (%) | High Risk n (%) |
|---|---|---|---|
| Sequence generation | 6 (50) | 6 (50) | 0 (0) |
| Allocation concealment | 0 (0) | 12 (100) | 0 (0) |
| Blinding of participants | 0 (0) | 1 (8.3) | 11 (91.7) |
| Blinding of personnel | 0 (0) | 1 (8.3) | 11 (91.7) |
| Blinding of outcome assessors | 0 (0) | 1 (8.3) | 11 (91.7) |
| Incomplete outcome data | 12 (100) | 0 (0) | 0 (0) |
| Selective outcome reporting | 0 (0) | 12 (100) | 0 (0) |

# Clinical Evidence for Combination Therapies from Randomised Controlled Trials

## Acupuncture plus Chinese Herbal Medicine vs. Antidepressants

Seven RCTs compared the effect of acupuncture plus CHM to anti-depressants alone (C4–C7, C10–C12). Meta-analysis was possible for five studies and the results showed significant improvement in Hamilton Rating Scale for Depression (HRSD) scores (standardised mean difference (SMD): –0.96 [–1.65, –0.27], $I^2$ = 89.2%) (Table 9.2). However, heterogeneity was "high". Selective serotonin reuptake inhibitor (SSRI) antidepressants were used as comparators in all studies and study duration ranged from four to 12 weeks. Meta-analysis was possible for three RCTs that assessed HRSD-24 scores. The results showed significant improvement in the HRSD-24 scores (MD: –2.81 [–4.61, –1.01], $I^2$ = 93.5%).

One study evaluated menopausal depression (C12). The mean HRSD-24 score significantly improved after acupuncture plus CHM was compared to antidepressants (MD: –7.33 [–12.22, –2.44]). One study (C10) assessed the Zung Self-rating Depression Scale (SDS) scores. Acupuncture in combination with CHM did not significantly improve SDS scores in 70 patients after eight weeks of treatment (MD: –0.79 [–2.64, 1.06]).

Two studies (C5, C6) reported on adverse events (AEs). In the treatment group, one study reported no AEs, whilst one study reported AEs such as headache (2 cases), reduced sleep time (1), and diarrhoea (1). In the antidepressant groups, AEs reported included drowsiness (6 cases), dry mouth (8), excessive sweating (5), reduced sleep time (2), dizziness (4), diarrhoea (4), and headache (4).

## Acupuncture plus Chinese Herbal Medicine vs. Placebo

Two RCTs studied the effect of acupuncture plus CHM, compared to placebo CHM (C6, C7). In 194 participants, four episodes of needle

**Table 9.2.    Evidence for Combination Therapies from Randomised Controlled Trials**

| Intervention | Comparator | Outcome | No. of Studies (Participants) | Effect Size (MD or SMD) [95% CI], I²%) | Included Studies |
|---|---|---|---|---|---|
| Acupuncture + Chinese herbal medince | Antidepressant | HRSD (all versions) | 5 (352) | SMD: −0.96 [−1.65, −0.27], I² = 89.2% | C3, C5, C9–C11 |
| | | HRSD-24 | 3 (222) | MD: −2.81 [−4.61, −1.01], I² = 93.5% | C4, C5, C11 |
| | | SDS | 1 (70) | MD: −0.79 [−2.64, 1.06] | C10 |
| Acupuncture + tuina 推拿 | Antidepressant | HRSD-24 | 1 (72) | MD: −3.11 [−5.62, −0.60]* | C8 |
| Acupuncture + moxibustion | Antidepressant | HRSD-24 | 1 (40) | MD: −5.44 [−8.39, −2.49]* | C1 |
| Acupuncture + moxibustion + five-element music therapy | Antidepressant | HRSD-24 | 1 (60) | MD: −1.6 [−4.81, 1.61] | C9 |
| Acupuncture + mobile cupping + psychotherapy | Psychotherapy | HRSD-17 | 1 (232) | MD: −4.28[−5.27, −3.29]* | C2 |
| Qigong 气功, tuina 推拿, and taichi 太极 + antidepressants | Antidepressant | HRSD | 1 (60) | MD: −11.33 [−16.3, −6.36]* | C3 |

* Statistically significant.

Abbreviations: HRSD, Hamilton Rating Scale for Depression; MD, mean difference; SMD, standardised mean difference fainting were reported. Other outcome measures did not meet the prespecified criteria and were not included in the analysis.

## Acupuncture plus *Tuina* vs. Antidepressants

One RCT assessed acupuncture plus *tuina* 推拿 compared with fluoxetine (C8). Acupuncture plus *tuina* 推拿 significantly improved the HRSD-24 score, compared to fluoxetine, in 72 participants after 40 days of treatment (MD: −3.11 [−5.62, −0.60]). The study did not report on AEs.

## Acupuncture plus Moxibustion vs. Antidepressants

One RCT compared acupuncture plus moxibustion to fluoxetine for depression during menopause (C1). Acupuncture plus moxibustion significantly improved the HRSD-24 score, compared to fluoxetine, in 40 participants after eight weeks of treatment (MD: −5.44 [−8.39, −2.49]). The study did not report on AEs.

## Acupuncture plus Moxibustion Plus Five-element Music Therapy vs. Antidepressants

One RCT compared acupuncture plus moxibustion and five-element music therapy to antidepressants (C9). However, the HRSD-24 score was not statistically significant between groups in 60 participants after six weeks of treatment (MD: −1.6 [−4.81, 1.61]). The study did not report on AEs.

## Acupuncture plus Cupping Plus Psychotherapy vs. Psychotherapy

One RCT studied the effect of acupuncture in combination with mobile cupping and psychotherapy (C2). The combination therapy improved the HRSD-17 score significantly, compared to antidepressants, in 232 participants after four weeks of treatment (MD: −4.28[−5.27, −3.29]). The study did not report on AEs.

## Qigong, Tuina, and Taichi plus Antidepressants vs. Antidepressants

One RCT combined *qigong* 气功, *tuina* 推拿, and *taichi* 太极 plus antidepressants with antidepressants alone (C3). The combination therapies significantly improved the HRSD score, compared to antidepressants, in 60 participants after 12 weeks of treatment (MD: –11.33 [–16.3, –6.36]). The study did not report on AEs.

# Controlled Clinical Trials of Combination Therapies

No non-randomised controlled clinical trials of combination therapies for depression were identified.

# Non-controlled Studies of Combination Therapies

Two studies were identified as non-controlled trials of combination therapies (C13, C14). A total of 74 participants were included in the studies. One study (C14) assessed the effect of CHM plus acupuncture for depression in people with Liver *qi* stagnation transforming into fire syndrome. One study (C13) assessed the effects of CHM combined with electroacupuncture. The studies did not report on AEs. The authors of both studies reported that the combination therapies improved depression.

## Summary of Combination Therapies

Various CM therapies are used together for the treatment of depression. The most common combination is CHM plus acupuncture, suggesting that this might be commonly used in clinical practice. It is interesting that one study assessed five-element music therapy for depression. However, more investigation is needed to determine its benefits. Acupuncture, in combination with CHM, *tuina* 推拿, moxibustion, and mobile cupping, showed beneficial effects for HRSD scores. However, the study numbers and sample sizes were small, and many studies did not report on AEs. Overall, there is insufficient evidence for the efficacy and safety of combination therapies of CM for the treatment of depression.

## References for Included Combination Therapies: Clinical Studies

| Study No. | References |
|---|---|
| C1 | 白艳甫, 杨帆. 针刺四关配合艾灸百会治疗围绝经期妇女抑郁症20例疗效观察.云南中医中药杂志, 2016, **37**(04): 45–46. |
| C2 | 曹辰虹, 陈静. 以督脉为主治疗抑郁症116例. 辽宁中医杂志, 2013, **40**(08): 1682–1684. |
| C3 | 谷建云, 成建平. 中医养生疗法辅助治疗抑郁症的临床疗效评价. 中国中医基础医学杂志, 2013, **19**(09): 1057–1059. |
| C4 | 吕沛宛, 郑伟锋. 针药并用疏肝解郁法治疗抑郁症的临床观察. 中国中医基础医学杂志, 2011, **17**(09): 1010–1011. |
| C5 | 邵妍. 针刺配合中药治疗抑郁症疗效观察. 辽宁中医药大学, 2008. |
| C6 | 徐峰. 逍遥散配合针灸治疗产后抑郁症的临床研究. 世界中西医结合杂志, 2013, **8**(09): 896–899. |
| C7 | 许芳, 唐启盛, 李小黎. 益肾调气法治疗产后抑郁症的随机对照临床研究. 北京中医药, 2013, **32**(03): 200–203. |
| C8 | 姚成龙. 针刺配合头面部推拿治疗肝郁气滞型抑郁症的临床研究. 长春中医药大学, 2014. |
| C9 | 张海兰, 王晓红. 五音疗法联合针刺、艾灸治疗肝气郁结型抑郁症随机平行对照研究. 实用中医内科杂志, 2016, **30**(01): 90–92. |
| C10 | 张永雷, 隋丽萍. 龟龙饮联合针刺对抑郁症患者血浆5-羟色胺含量的影响. 国际中医中药杂志, 2013, **35**(04): 303–305. |
| C11 | 周秀芳, 胡捷, 张迎梅, 陈河燕. 附子逍遥散配合快速针刺法治疗抑郁症的临床观察. 中国药房, 2016, **27**(11): 1515–1517. |
| C12 | 朱慧玲. 针药结合治疗肝郁肾虚型围绝经期抑郁症的临床观察. 黑龙江中医药大学, 2013. |
| C13 | 褚丽丽, 邢艳丽. 针药结合治疗肝郁化火型抑郁症40例. 针灸临床杂志, 2009, **25**(08): 14–15. |
| C14 | 金成, 刘晓芳. 电针加逍遥丸治疗慢性抑郁症34例疗效观察. 现代中医药, 2007(05): 73. |

# 10

# Summary and Conclusions

## OVERVIEW

This chapter summarises the main findings of the previous chapters, including those from the classical literature, clinical trial evidence, and experimental evidence. Chinese medicine therapies, including herbal medicine and acupuncture, are discussed regarding the clinical management of depression. Limitations of the available evidence are reported, and future directions identified for clinical and experimental research.

## Introduction

Chinese medicine (CM) therapies are used as a part of the management of depression, often in combination with pharmacotherapies and psychotherapy. Current conventional management of depression has three treatment phases and ongoing monitoring. Acute treatment aims to induce remission and achieve full return of the patient's level of functioning to that experienced prior to the depressive episode. The continuation phase aims to reduce relapse and the maintenance phase may, or may not, require ongoing treatment depending on each patient's circumstances. During the maintenance phase patients are monitored for potential relapse.[1,2]

Most patients are given second-generation antidepressants such as selective serotonin reuptake inhibitors (SSRIs), which are optimal in terms of safety and efficacy.[3] However, side effects have been reported across different antidepressant drugs, including dizziness and sweating (tricyclic antidepressants and norepinephrine reuptake inhibitors), gastrointestinal and sexual side effects (SSRIs), and sedation and weight gain (noradrenergic and specific serotonergic antidepressants).[4] Non-pharmacological treatments, such as psychotherapy and electro-convulsive therapy, are also available and have positive effects but the results vary between individual patients. Clinically, depression is a lifelong and recurrent disease and current therapies have limited efficacy and are not curative. Consequently, complementary and alternative therapies, such as CM, can be considered in the overall management of depression.

This monograph includes a "whole-evidence" analysis of CM for the management of depression. A review of clinical guidelines and textbooks have identified the main syndromes for depression and recommended CM treatments, including oral Chinese herbal medicine (CHM) and acupuncture (Chapter 2). Review of the classical literature identified traditional use of herbal medicine (Chapter 3). Numerous clinical trials reveal the promising benefits of oral CHM for depression (Chapter 5). Current available pre-clinical evidence has also been reviewed to explain the probable mechanisms of action of the commonly used herbs (Chapter 6). There are a limited number of acupuncture studies for depression, but the available evidence suggests benefit (Chapter 7). Only two studies have evaluated *tuina* 推拿 and cupping for depression and further research is warranted (Chapter 8). The combination of CHM plus acupuncture was evaluated in multiple studies with some evidence of benefit (Chapter 9).

## Chinese Medicine Syndrome Differentiation

Current clinical guidelines categorise depression into six syndromes according to the presenting signs and symptoms. For each syndrome, a single formula or combined formulae are suggested as a guide for clinical practice (Chapter 2). In the classical literature (Chapter 3), there was an emphasis on depression being caused by emotional disturbance leading to an imbalance of the *zang fu* organs, with the Heart being impaired. Citations often suggested depression is caused by *qi* and phlegm stagnation or *qi* deficiency.

Most CHM clinical studies did not specify the use of CM syndromes for selection of CHM interventions for depression, but a few studies did use syndrome differentiation as inclusion criteria or as criteria for selecting the formula used. The most common syndromes were generally consistent with those mentioned in the clinical practice guidelines (Chapter 2), although there were some differences. In studies that described CM syndromes, the common syndromes included Liver *qi* stagnation, Heart and Spleen deficiency, Liver *qi* stagnation with Spleen deficiency, *qi* stagnation transforming into heat, phlegm stagnation, melancholy disturbing the mind, and the Heart and Kidneys not interacting.

In the 56 studies on acupuncture and related therapies, only 14 studies used syndrome differentiation. The most commonly reported syndrome was Liver *qi* stagnation. Other syndromes included Heart and Spleen deficiency, Liver *qi* stagnation with Spleen deficiency, *qi* stagnation transforming into heat, phlegm stagnation, and melancholy disturbing the mind. Studies assessing other CM therapies did not mention syndrome differentiation. Five out of 12 combination CM therapy studies mentioned syndrome differentiation. Only one study used syndrome differentiation to select acupuncture points, others selected study participants using syndrome differentiation.

Syndrome differentiation could not be used as a classifying factor to pool studies and analyse whether a particular syndrome was more or less effective in producing a positive effect in the clinical studies. This was due to the small number of studies that reported syndromes and the large number of different syndromes. In the studies that used treatments based on syndrome differentiation the results were presented as aggregates so further analysis was not possible.

# Chinese Herbal Medicine

In total, 121 clinical studies evaluated CHM for depression. Most studies were randomised controlled trials (RCTs) and compared CHM to antidepressants, or administered a combination of CHM and antidepressants, compared to antidepressants alone. All the CHM interventions were orally administrated. Of the antidepressants, SSRIs were the most frequently used.

A considerable number of instruments measured depression severity. The instruments with sufficient data suitable for pooling were the Hamilton Rating Scale for Depression (HRSD), Zung's Self-rating Depression Scale (SDS), Montgomery–Asberg Depression Rating Scale (MADRS) and the Edinburgh Postnatal Depression Scale (EPDS). Other outcomes, such as relapse and remission of depression, quality of life, functional capacity, and suicidality were not commonly used. Most studies provided data after one to 12 weeks of treatment.

Chinese herbal medicine reduced depression severity, compared to placebo, measured by the HRSD and the EPDS. Despite the positive results there were a limited number of studies with small sample sizes. Meta-analysis also showed CHM reduced depression severity, compared with antidepressants. However, included studies were not free of bias. Considerable heterogeneity was also noted and could not be identified by subgroup analysis. Variable aetiologies, severity of depression, disease history, and different CHM interventions in terms of treatment duration, ingredients, dosage, and medication compliance may be the cause of heterogeneity. Chinese herbal medicine showed the largest effect when administered for six weeks or less. This may indicate a strong placebo effect in the participants or that the time course of effect is short. Chinese herbal medicine also showed significant benefit for women with postpartum depression and menopausal depression, compared to antidepressants.

When CHM was combined with antidepressants (integrative medicine), the pooled results showed the addition of CHM produced more benefits than antidepressants alone in terms of reducing depression severity based on the HRSD, SDS, MADRS, and EPDS. Despite the positive results there was considerable heterogeneity, which might be due to inconsistency across studies in terms of depression aetiology, disease history, different herbal formulae, treatment durations, and outcome measurements. In terms of the HRSD scores, heterogeneity was reduced by subgrouping different versions of the HRSD. Integrative medicine also reduced depression severity in women with postpartum depression but not menopausal depression.

However, only one study with a small sample size was available to assess the efficacy of CHM for menopausal depression.

Compared with psychotherapy, CHM plus psychotherapy was superior in terms of improving depression symptoms, as was CHM plus antidepressants plus psychotherapy, compared to antidepressants and psychotherapy. However, study numbers and sample sizes were small, therefore the meta-analysis results indicated that the additional benefit brought by integrative medicine, compared to antidepressants and/or psychotherapy, remains unclear and further high-quality studies are needed.

Regarding safety, participants taking CHM reported similar AEs as those taking a placebo. The total AEs in the CHM groups, either CHM alone or integrative CHM, was less than that in the control groups.

## Chinese Herbal Medicine Formulae in Key Clinical Guidelines and Textbooks, Classical Literature and Clinical Studies

This section summarises the evidence from Chapters 2, 3 and 5. Overall, the CHM used for depression is consistent between classical literature, contemporary clinical practice guidelines, and clinical trials (Table 10.1). Thirteen formulae were specified in Chapter 2 based on CM syndrome differentiation. These are generally consistent with the most frequently used formulae in the classic literature including: *Gan mai da zao tang* 甘麦大枣汤, *Xiao yao san/wan* 逍遥散汤/丸, *Gui pi tang/wan* 归脾汤/丸, and *Qi fu yin* 七福饮. Out of these, *Qi fu yin* 七福饮, which is used for deficiency of *qi* and Blood, did not appear in key guidelines, textbooks, or clinical trials. This is likely to be, because contemporary CM practitioners use *Gui pi tang/wan* 归脾汤/丸 as a standard formula for depression caused by deficiency of the Heart and Spleen. The common formulae in the clinical trials were *Chai hu shu gan san* 柴胡疏肝散, *Xiao yao san/wan* 逍遥散, *Dan zhi xiao yao san* 丹栀逍遥散, *An shen ding zhi tang* 安神定志汤, *Bu shen shu gan hua yu tang* 补肾疏肝化瘀汤, and *Jia wei xiao yao capsules* 加味逍遥胶囊.

**Table 10.1. Summary of Chinese Herbal Medicine Formulae**

| Formula Name | Included in Clinical Guidelines and Textbooks | Included in Classical Literature (No. of Citations) | Included in Clinical Studies (Chapter 5) | | | Included in Combination Therapies (Chapter 9) |
|---|---|---|---|---|---|---|
| | | | RCTs (No. of Studies) | CCTs (No. of Studies) | Non-controlled Studies (No. of Studies) | |
| Ban xia hou po tang 半夏厚朴汤 | Yes | 0 | 1 | 0 | 1 | 0 |
| Chai hu shu gan san 柴胡疏肝散 | Yes | 0 | 3 | 1 | 3 | 0 |
| Dan zhi xiao yao san 丹栀逍遥散 | Yes | 0 | 3 | 0 | 1 | 0 |
| Gan mai da zao tang 甘麦大枣汤 | Yes | 63 | 0 | 0 | 0 | 0 |
| Gui pi tang/wan 归脾汤/丸 | Yes | 33 | 1 | 0 | 0 | 0 |
| Liu wei di huang wan 六味地黄丸 | Yes | 0 | 0 | 0 | 0 | 0 |
| Long dan xie gan tang 龙胆泻肝汤 | Yes | 2 | 0 | 0 | 0 | 0 |
| Si ni san 四逆散 | Yes | 0 | 0 | 0 | 0 | 0 |
| Tian wan bu xin dan 天王补心丹 | Yes | 0 | 0 | 0 | 0 | 0 |
| Tong qiao huo xue tang 通窍活血汤 | Yes | 0 | 0 | 0 | 0 | 0 |
| Wen dan tang 温胆汤 | Yes | 7 | 0 | 0 | 0 | 0 |
| Xiao yao san/wan 逍遥散汤/丸 | Yes | 8 | 4 | 0 | 0 | 1 |
| Xue Fu Zhu Yu Tang 血府逐瘀汤 | Yes | 0 | 0 | 0 | 0 | 0 |
| Yue ju wan 越鞠丸 | Yes | 3 | 1 | 0 | 0 | 0 |
| Zi shui qing gan yin 滋水清肝饮 | Yes | 0 | 0 | 0 | 0 | 0 |
| An shen ding zhi tang 安神定志汤 | No | 0 | 0 | 0 | 0 | 0 |
| Bu shen shu gan hua yu tang 补肾疏肝化瘀汤 | No | 0 | 2 | 0 | 0 | 0 |
| Jia wei xiao yao capsules 加味逍遥胶囊 | No | 0 | 2 | 0 | 0 | 0 |
| Qi fu yin 七福饮 | No | 8 | 0 | 0 | 0 | 0 |

*Note:* The total number of studies in each section included: 319 classical literature citations, 104 RCTs, 4 CCTs, and 13 non-controlled studies.

Abbreviations: CCTs, controlled clinical trials; RCTs, randomised controlled trials.

A few formulae found in contemporary clinical guidelines, have not been investigated in clinical studies and classical literature, these include: *Xue fu zhu yu tang* 血府逐瘀汤, *Tong qiao huo xue tang* 通窍活血, *Si ni san* 四逆散, *Long dan xie gan tang* 龙胆泻肝汤, *Zi shui qing gan yin* 滋水清肝饮, *Tian wang bu xin dan* 天王补心丹, and *Liu wei di huang wan* 六味地黄丸. This may be due to current clinical trials focusing on the short-term pathogenesis of depression, including Liver *qi* stagnation. However, long-term pathogenesis may include stagnant *qi* transforming into phlegm, Blood stasis, or damp-heat in the Liver meridian. The guideline recommended formulae are used for later stage depression based on the clinical experience of CM practitioners.

*Wan dan tang* 温胆汤 and *Long dan xie gan tang* 龙胆泻肝汤 were found in contemporary clinical guidelines and classical literature but were not included in clinical studies. This is mainly because these studies did not meet the inclusion criteria and used outcomes that were not pre-specified or controls that were not standard treatments. Out of all the formulae evaluated in clinical trials, *Chai hu shu gan san* 柴胡疏肝散, *Xiao yao san* 逍遥散, *Dan zhi xiao yao san* 丹栀逍遥散, *Gui pi tang* 归脾汤, *Ban xia hou po tang* 半夏厚朴汤 and *Yue ju wan* 越鞠丸 were recommended in contemporary clinical guidelines.

The most commonly used formula in clinical trials was *Chai hu shu gan san* 柴胡疏肝散, which appeared in three RCTs, one controlled clinical trial (CCT) and three non-controlled studies. *Chai hu shu gan san* 柴胡疏肝散, either used alone or combined with antidepressants, showed benefits in terms of reducing depression severity on the HRSD scale when compared with antidepressants alone. *Chai hu shu gan san* 柴胡疏肝散 is also recommended in contemporary clinical practice guidelines for Liver *qi* depression syndrome. However, it was not found in the classical literature for depression, likely because the formula was originally used for subcostal pain, not depression, as stated in the book *Zhen zhi zhun sheng* 证治准绳 (1368–1644 A.D).

The next most frequently researched formula was *Xiao yao san/ wan* 逍遥散, which appeared in four RCTs. It reduced HRSD score indicating less depression severity. *Dan zhi xiao yao san* 丹栀逍遥散,

which was used in three RCTs and one non-controlled study, did not show benefits in terms of the HRSD and SDS but appeared to be safe. *Xiao yao san/wan* 逍遥散 was commonly cited in the classical literature citations and is also recommended in the contemporary clinical practice guidelines.

A few manufactured products, such as *Shu gan jie yu* capsules 舒肝解郁胶囊 and *Ba ji tian gua tang* capsules 巴戟天寡糖胶囊 are recommend in clinical guidelines and found in clinical studies. These products have also been approved by the China Food and Drug Administration. *Shu gan jie yu* capsules 舒肝解郁胶囊 are St. John's Wort extracts used in CM and Western herbal medicine. Despite the current clinical trial research, more high-quality RCTs are needed to further confirm their efficacy and safety.

Overall, CHM showed promising effects and was safe for depression. However, interpretation of the results should consider relatively poor methodological quality of the studies including a general lack of blinding of participants and personnel, small sample sizes, and heterogeneity. These aspects reduce confidence in the results and led to the downgrading of the quality of the evidence in the Grading of Recommendations Assessment, Development and Evaluation (GRADE) assessments (Chapter 5: Tables 5.4 and 5.5).

## Acupuncture and Related Therapies

This section summarises the evidence from Chapters 2, 3 and 7. The clinical guidelines (Chapter 2) recommend manual acupuncture using a few main acupuncture points based on syndrome differentiation. Few citations in the classical literature reported acupuncture and moxibustion for depression (Chapter 3). Out of the 56 acupuncture clinical studies, the majority evaluated the effects of manual acupuncture or electroacupuncture for depression. There were no CCTs. The acupuncture therapies recommended in Chapter 2 and found in Chapter 3, have also been studied in multiple RCTs and are listed in Table 10.2. A number of CM syndromes have been reported in clinical studies, which overlap with syndromes recommended in guidelines and textbooks and classical literature. Liver *qi* stagnation,

**Table 10.2. Summary of Acupuncture and Related Therapies**

| Intervention | Included in Clinical Guidelines and Textbooks (Chapter 2) | Included in Classical Literature (Chapter 3) (No. of Citations) | Included in Clinical Studies (Chapter 7) | | | Included in Combination Therapies (Chapter 9) |
|---|---|---|---|---|---|---|
| | | | RCTs (No. of Studies) | CCTs (No. of Studies) | Non-controlled Studies* (No. of Studies) | |
| Acupuncture | Yes | 5 | 33 | NA | 6 | 12 |
| Electroacupuncture | No | 0 | 16 | NA | 2 | 0 |
| Non-penetrating acupoint stimulation (TENS or laser) | No | 0 | 3 | NA | 0 | 0 |
| Moxibustion | No | 3 | 0 | NA | 0 | 1 |
| **Acupuncture Points** | | | | | | |
| HT7 Shenmen 神门 | Yes | 0 | 11 | NA | 3 | 7 |
| PC7 Daling 大陵 | Yes | 1 | 2 | NA | 0 | 0 |
| PC6 Neiguan 内关 | Yes | 1 | 23 | NA | 6 | 9 |
| LR14 Qimen 期门 | Yes | 0 | 3 | NA | 0 | 3 |
| HT15 Xinshu 心俞 | Yes | 1 | 6 | NA | 0 | 2 |
| LI4 Hegu 合谷 | Yes | 0 | 8 | NA | 0 | 2 |
| LR3 Taichong 太冲 | Yes | 0 | 17 | NA | 3 | 9 |
| PC5 Jianshi 间使 | No | 1 | 1 | NA | 0 | 0 |
| KI6 Zhaohai 照海 | No | 1 | 1 | NA | 0 | 0 |
| GV20 Baihui 百会 | No | 0 | 35 | NA | 6 | 10 |
| EX-HN3 Yintang 印堂 | No | 0 | 22 | NA | 3 | 5 |
| BL18 Ganshu 肝俞 | Yes | 0 | 13 | NA | 1 | 3 |
| SP6 Sanyinjiao 三阴交 | Yes | 0 | 15 | NA | 0 | 3 |

*Some studies used more than one intervention e.g. acupuncture plus moxibustion. They are counted separately in this table.

Note: The total number of studies in each section included: 9 classical literature citations, 48 RCTs, 0 CCTs, and 8 non-controlled studies.

Abbreviations: CCTs, controlled clinical trials; NA, not applicable; RCTs, Randomised controlled trials; TENS, transcutaneous electrical nerve stimulation.

Heart and Spleen deficiency, Liver *qi* stagnation with Spleen deficiency were common across all types of literature.

Acupoints PC6 *Neiguan* 内关, PC7 *Daling* 大陵 and HT15 *Xinshu* 心俞 were points described in the classical, contemporary and clinical study literature. Some frequently used points in clinical studies also included GV20 *Baihui* 百会, PC6 *Neiguan* 内关, EX-HN3 *Yintang* 印堂, LR3 *Taichong* 太冲, HT7 *Shenmen* 神门. and SP6 *Sanyinjiao* 三阴交. Acupoint LR3 *Taichong* 太冲 is recommended in the clinical guidelines but was not mentioned in classical literature. Acupoints PC5 *Jianshi* 间使 and KI6 *Zhaohai* 照海 are described in classical literature and evaluated in one clinical study, but not recommended in clinical guidelines. Only eight citations relating to acupuncture therapies were identified in the classical literature, therefore this may affect the point comparisons.

Evidence from acupuncture RCTs showed a reduction in depression severity, when used alone or in combination with antidepressants. Two studies reported on health-related quality of life, however, the results were inconclusive. Few AEs from acupuncture therapies were reported when acupuncture therapies were assessed alone. When evaluated in combination with antidepressants, the number of AEs increased. In combination therapy studies, that is CHM plus acupuncture, meta-analysis showed significant improvement in the HRSD scores, but heterogeneity was present. For other CM therapy combinations, evidence is only available from single studies. Therefore, it is difficult to draw a reliable conclusion on the efficacy and safety of combination therapies for depression.

## Other Chinese Medicine Therapies

This section summarises the evidence from Chapters 2, 3 and 8. The guidelines recommended diet therapy for depression: congees using foods that have *qi* tonifying and calming the mind properties. There was no mention of diet therapy in classical literature or clinical studies. Limited clinical trial evidence on other CM therapies was found. Chapter 8 presented evidence of mobile cupping therapy and *tuina* 推拿 for depression (Table 10.3). Mobile cupping was along the

**Table 10.3.  Summary of Other Chinese Medicine Therapies**

| Intervention | Included in Clinical Guidelines and Textbooks (Chapter 2) | Included in Classical Literature (Chapter 3) (No. of Citations) | Included in Clinical Studies (Chapter 8) | | | Included in Combination Therapies (Chapter 9) |
|---|---|---|---|---|---|---|
| | | | RCTs (No. of Studies) | CCTs (No. of Studies) | Non-controlled Studies (No. of Studies) | |
| Cupping | No | No | 1 | NA | NA | Yes |
| Tuina 推拿 | No | No | 1 | NA | NA | Yes |
| Diet therapy | Yes | No | 0 | NA | NA | No |

*Note:* The total number of studies in each section included: 0 classical literature citations, 2 RCTs, 0 CCTs, and 0 non-controlled studies.

Abbreviations: CCTs, controlled clinical trials; RCTs, randomised controlled trials; NA, not applicable.

governor vessel and bladder meridians, *tuina* 推拿 was performed on acupoints including HT7 *Shenmen* 神门, PC8 *Laogong* 劳宫, KI3 *Taixi* 太溪, ST36 *Zusanli* 足三里, and BL15 *Xinshu* 心俞. Some points used in the *tuina* 推拿 study overlapped with the most frequently used acupuncture points in acupuncture clinical studies (Table 10.2). Both studies showed significant improvements in HRSD-24 scores. One study, using mobile cupping in combination with antidepressants, reported similar AEs in both groups.

Overall, there were only two clinical studies of other CM therapies for depression. The available studies were not blinded and there was inadequacies in the reporting of study methods. Due to the small number of studies and poor methodological quality, it was not possible to conclude the effectiveness and safety of these therapies.

## Limitations of Evidence

Significant effort was made to collect and analyse data from a range of sources, yet omissions from each of the data sets are possible. The overview of current CM clinical practice in Chapter 2, are taken from authoritative clinical practice guidelines and textbooks. However, this is not a comprehensive list and some syndromes and treatments which are not widely used are not included in Chapter 2. In addition, recommendations may change in the future.

The classical literature in Chapter 3 is a comprehensive summary of the treatment of depression in ancient times. However, the literature was only from one source, the Encyclopedia of Chinese Medicine (Zhong Hua Yi Dian, ZHYD). The ZHYD is the largest searchable resource, but it does not contain every historical CM text and some classical books may have been missed. Twenty search terms were used to find the depression citations, yet searching more terms may have found more citations. In terms of the search results, there was only a very small number of acupuncture citations and it is unknown if acupuncture was seldom used in ancient times or relevant citations were inadvertently omitted from the search.

Clinical trial evidence presented in Chapters 5, 7–9 includes literature from a comprehensive search of the Chinese and English scientific databases. However, errors or misclassification may have occurred during the screening process. When appropriate, meta-analysis was conducted to provide aggregate data from multiple studies. The evidence for CM interventions, compared to placebo or conventional treatments such as antidepressants and psychotherapy, showed consistent results in favour of CHM/acupuncture or integrative medicine (CHM/acupuncture plus antidepressants). Of studies included in meta-analyses, variations such as demographic features, depression aetiology, comorbidity and outcome measurements were considerable. Consequently, substantial statistical heterogeneity was observed in pooled results that could not be explained by subgroup analysis. To account for the heterogeneity a random effects model was used to provide conservative estimations of effect sizes.

In addition, most studies had methodological shortfalls including insufficient random allocation procedures, lack of blinding of participants and personnel and small sample sizes. Furthermore the main outcome, the HRSD, lacked version consistency amongst the studies and the version was not always specified. These methodological shortfalls and insufficient reporting in the published manuscripts compromised the results, leading to downgrading of the evidence quality. Furthermore, adverse events were insufficiently reported.

Studies evaluating depression subgroups, such as postpartum depression and menopausal depression, were few in number and a firm conclusion could not be drawn from the current clinical evidence. Compared with psychotherapy alone, the addition of CHM or acupuncture was superior in terms of improving depression symptoms. However, there were only a small number of studies with small sample sizes and the true effect remains unclear. Limited clinical evidence of other CM therapies, such as *tuina* 推拿 and cupping, was available for synthesis. Studies that used *taichi* 太极 and *qigong* 气功 were excluded due to the age restriction of the monograph inclusion criteria.

Chinese herbal medicine and acupuncture given together was assessed in a small number of clinical studies and different herbs and acupuncture points were used in the studies. Therefore, it was difficult to draw a firm conclusion on their efficacy for depression. The limitations discussed above should be taken into consideration when interpreting the results in this monograph.

# Implications for Practice

A summary of information from the clinical guidelines and textbooks (Chapter 2) provides important guidance for syndrome differentiation and selection of appropriate CM treatments for people with depression. Depression is a condition that arises from emotional upset, overthinking or excess worry. The main organs involved are the Liver, Heart, Spleen and Kidney. Liver *qi* stagnation has been described across contemporary, classical and clinical trial evidence and should be considered the main syndrome for depression. Chinese herbal medicine or acupuncture alone, or combined with antidepressants, improve depression severity. Other CM therapies such as *tuina* 推拿, cupping, *taichi* 太极 and *qigong* 气功 are not found in contemporary or classical literature and not commonly researched. The most commonly studied herbs with a favourable effect for depression are *chai hu* 柴胡, *shao yao* 芍药, *gan cao* 甘草, *yuan zhi* 远志, and *shi chang pu* 石菖蒲. The most commonly studied acupuncture points with a favourable effect are: GV20

*Baihui* 百会, EX-HN3 *Yintang* 印堂, PC6 *Neiguan* 内关, LR3 *Taichong* 太冲, and SP6 *Sanyinjiao* 三阴交.

In the CHM studies the largest effect was observed with treatment duration of six weeks or less. This may indicate a strong placebo effect in these participants or the time course of effect is short. The observation is different in acupuncture studies; RCTs comparing acupuncture to antidepressants with treatment duration of more than six weeks showed significant effects on reducing depression severity. Taken together, these findings indicate CHM and acupuncture are effective at reducing depression severity and could be considered as part of an overall treatment plan for people with depression.

## Implications for Research

Many clinical studies evaluated the effect and safety of CM therapies for depression. Encouraging evidence is available for CHM and acupuncture therapies but evidence is lacking for other therapies. Further research will increase knowledge and help to improve the management of depression. Despite the common use of several herbs in clinical studies, preclinical studies relevant to depression were limited, especially for *fu ling* 茯苓, *dang gui* 当归, *yu jin* 郁金, *bai zhu* 白术, *suan zao ren* 酸枣仁, *xiang fu* 香附, *chuan xiong* 川芎, *chen pi* 陈皮, *zhi zi* 栀子, *he huan pi* 合欢皮, and *dang shen* 党参. Future experimental studies will improve the understanding of their mechanisms of action and may lead to new therapeutic agents.

Rigorous methodology is needed when designing future clinical trials of CM therapies for depression. Methods of sequence generation and allocation concealment should be clearly stated. Due to the nature of acupuncture practice, blinding of personnel is difficult in acupuncture studies. However, this was possible in three studies that used sham electroacupuncture or laser equipment. Sham acupuncture needles could be used in future studies to improve the blinding of personnel and reduce the risk of bias. Future RCTs should have their protocols published and be registered to minimise reporting bias and increase transparency in the reporting of the results.

Cause of disease, depression severity and disease course should be taken into consideration when designing trials; more comparable and reliable results will be produced if similar participants are recruited. A considerable number of depression severity instruments were reported as main outcome measures, such as the HRSD, SDS, MADRS, and the EPDS. But other clinically important outcomes were not, such as relapse and remission of depression, quality of life, functional capacity, and suicidality. Assessing these outcomes would provide a better understanding of the effect of CM therapies for depression.

The majority of clinical trials included treatment for one to 12 weeks and only a few reported follow-up data. Depression is a lifelong disease and follow-up assessment would provide long-term evidence of CM therapies for depression and further strengthen the evidence. Most studies did not specify the use of CM syndromes for selection of CHM or acupuncture interventions. Where possible, CM treatments should be given based on syndrome differentiation. This will validate CM theory and improve translation of results into clinical practice.

The majority of RCTs included in this monograph were assessed as "unclear" risk of bias for many domains due to insufficiency of the details provided. Future clinical studies should follow the items required by the Consolidated Standards of Reporting Trials (CONSORT)[5] and its extensions for herbal medicine, traditional CM and acupuncture.[6-9] Informative reporting of trial participants, reason for intervention selection, comparator, and results of validated outcome measures will provide high level clinical evidence and benefit practitioners, researchers and patients.

# References

1.  Gartlehner G, Gaynes B, Amick H, *et al.* (2015) Nonpharmacological Versus Pharmacological Treatments for Adult Patients With Major Depressive Disorder. Rockville (MD): Agency for Healthcare Research and Quality (USA).

2.  Kupfer DJ, Frank E and Phillips ML. (2012) Major depressive disorder: new clinical, neurobiological, and treatment perspectives. *Lancet* **379**(9820): 1045–1055.

3.  Practice guideline for the treatment of patients with major depressive disorder. (2000) American Psychiatric Association. *Am J Psychiatry* **157** (4 Suppl): 1–45.

4.  Anderson IM, Ferrier IN, Baldwin RC, *et al.* (2008) Evidence-based guidelines for treating depressive disorders with antidepressants: a revision of the 2000 British Association for Psychopharmacology guidelines. *J Psychopharmacol* **22**(4): 343–396.

5.  Schulz KF, Altman DG, Moher D, *et al.* (2010) CONSORT 2010 Statement: updated guidelines for reporting parallel group randomised trials. *Trials* 11.

6.  Gagnier JJ, Boon H, Rochon P, *et al.* (2006) Reporting randomized, controlled trials of herbal interventions: An elaborated CONSORT statement. *Ann Intern Med* **144**(5): 364–367.

7.  Bian Z, Liu B, Moher D, *et al.* (2011) Consolidated standards of reporting trials (CONSORT) for traditional Chinese medicine: current situation and future development. *Front Med* **5**(2): 171–177.

8.  MacPherson H, White A, Cummings M, *et al.* (2002) Standards for reporting interventions in controlled trials of acupuncture: The STRICTA recommendations. STandards for Reporting Interventions in Controlled Trails of Acupuncture. *Acupunct Med* **20**(1): 22–25.

9.  MacPherson H, Altman DG, Hammerschlag R, *et al.* (2010) Revised Standards for Reporting Interventions in Clinical Trials of Acupuncture (STRICTA): Extending the CONSORT statement. *J Evid Based Med* **3**(3): 140–155.

# Glossary

| Terms | Acronym | Definition | Reference |
|---|---|---|---|
| 95% confidence interval | 95% CI | A measure of the uncertainty around the main finding of a statistical analysis. Estimates of unknown quantities, such as the odds ratio comparing an experimental intervention with a control, are usually presented as a point estimate and a 95% confidence interval. This means that if someone were to keep repeating a study in other samples from the same population, 95% of the confidence intervals from those studies would contain the true value of the unknown quantity. Alternatives to 95%, such as 90% and 99% confidence intervals, are sometimes used. Wider intervals indicate lower precision; narrow intervals, greater precision. | http://handbook.cochrane.org/ |
| Acupuncture | — | The insertion of needles into humans or animals for remedial purposes or its methods. | WHO International Standard Terminologies of Traditional Medicine in the Western Pacific Region. World Health Organisation; 2007. |
| Allied and Complementary Medicine Database | AMED | Alternative medicine bibliographic database. | http://www.ovid.com/site/catalog/databases/l2.jsp |
| Australian New Zealand Clinical Trial Registry | ANZCTR | Australian clinical trial registry. | http://www.anzctr.org.au/ |
| Beck Depression Inventory | BDI | Questionnaire that rates the severity of depression. | Beck AT, Ward CH, Mendelson M, Mock J and Erbaugh J. (1961) An inventory for measuring |

(*Continued*)

(Continued)

| Terms | Acronym | Definition | Reference |
|---|---|---|---|
| | | | depression. *Arch Gen Psychiatry* **4**: 561–571. |
| China National Knowledge Infrastructure | CNKI | Chinese language bibliographic database. | http://www.cnki.net |
| Chinese Biomedical Literature Database | CBM | Chinese language bibliographic database. | http://www.imicams. ac.cn/ |
| Chinese Clinical Trial Registry | ChiCTR | Chinese clinical trial registry. | http://www.chictr.org/ |
| Chinese herbal medicine | CHM | Chinese herbal medicine. | — |
| Chinese medicine | CM | — | — |
| Chongqing VIP Information Company | CQVIP | Chinese language bibliographic database. | http://www.cqvip.com |
| ClinicalTrials.gov | — | Clinical trial registry. | https://clinicaltrials.gov/ |
| Cochrane Central Register of Controlled Trials | CENTRAL | Bibliographic database that provides a highly concentrated source of reports of controlled trials. | http://community. cochrane.org/editorial-and-publishing-policy-resource/ cochrane-central-register-controlled-trials-central |
| Combination therapies | — | Two or more Chinese medicines from different therapy groups (e.g. Chinese herbal medicine, acupuncture therapies or other Chinese medicine therapies) administered together. | — |
| Controlled clinical trials | CCT | An experimental study in which people are allocated to different interventions using methods that are not random. | http://handbook.cochrane. org/ |
| Convention on International Trade in Endangered Species of Wild Fauna and Flora | CITES | — | https://www.cites.org/eng/ disc/text.php |
| Cumulative Index of Nursing and Allied Health Literature | CINAHL | Bibliographic database. | https://www.ebscohost. com/nursing/about |
| Cupping therapy | — | Suction by using a vaccumised cup or jar. | WHO International Standard Terminologies of Traditional Medicine in the Western Pacific Region. World Health Organisation; 2007. |

## (*Continued*)

| Terms | Acronym | Definition | Reference |
|---|---|---|---|
| Diagnostic and Statistical Manual of Mental Disorders | DSM | American Psychiatric Association's diagnostic manual. | American Psychiatric Association. Diagnostic and Statistical Manual of Mental Disorders, 5th ed. American Psychiatric Association, Arlington, VA; 2013. |
| Disability adjusted life years | DALY | DALYs are a measurement of disease expressed in units. Years lived with disability are added to the number of years of life lost for a certain disease. | https://www.nimh.nih.gov/health/statistics/disability/what-are-ylds.shtml |
| Edinburgh Postnatal Depression Scale | EPDS | Questionnaire that rates the symptoms of postnatal depression. | Cox JL, Holden JM, and Sagovsky R. (1987) Detection of postnatal depression. Development of the 10-item Edinburgh Postnatal Depression Scale. *Br J Psychiatry* **150**: 782–786. |
| Effect size | — | A generic term for the estimate of effect of treatment for a study. | http://handbook.cochrane.org/ |
| Electroacupuncture | — | Electric stimulation of the needle following insertion. | WHO International Standard Terminologies of Traditional Medicine in the Western Pacific Region. World Health Organisation; 2007. |
| EU Clinical Trials Register | EU-CTR | European clinical trial registry. | https://www.clinicaltrialsregister.eu |
| Excerpta Medica database | Embase | Bibliographic database. | http://www.elsevier.com/solutions/embase |
| Grading of Recommendations Assessment, Development and Evaluation | GRADE | Approach used to grade quality of evidence and strength of recommendations. | http://www.gradeworkinggroup.org/ |
| Hamilton Rating Scale for Depression | HRSD | Questionnaire that rates the severity of depression. | Hamilton M. (1960) A rating scale for depression. *J Neurol Neurosurg Psychiatry* **23**(1): 56–62. |

(*Continued*)

## (Continued)

| Terms | Acronym | Definition | Reference |
|---|---|---|---|
| Heterogeneity | — | Used in a general sense to describe the variation in, or diversity of, participants, interventions, and measurement of outcomes across a set of studies, or the variation in internal validity of those studies. Used specifically, as statistical heterogeneity, to describe the degree of variation in the effect estimates from a set of studies. Also used to indicate the presence of variability among studies beyond the amount expected due solely to the play of chance. | http://handbook.cochrane.org/ |
| Homogeneity | — | Used in a general sense to mean that the participants, interventions, and measurement of outcomes are similar across a set of studies. Used specifically to describe the effect estimates from a set of studies where they do not vary more than would be expected by chance. | http://handbook.cochrane.org/ |
| $I^2$ | — | A measure of study heterogeneity, indicates the percentage of variance in a meta-analysis. | http://handbook.cochrane.org/ |
| Integrative medicine | — | Chinese herbal medicine combined with pharmacotherapy or other conventional therapy. | |
| International Classification of Diseases-10th Revision | ICD-10 | World Health Organisation's International Classification of Diseases | World Health Organisation. (1993) International Classification of Diseases (ICD-10) World Health Organisation, Geneva, Switzerland. |
| Mean difference | MD | In meta-analysis: A method used to combine measures on continuous scales, where the mean, standard deviation and sample size in each group are known. The weight given to the difference in means from each study (e.g. how much influence each study has on the overall results of the meta-analysis) is determined by the precision of its estimate of effect, | http://handbook.cochrane.org/ |

## (*Continued*)

| Terms | Acronym | Definition | Reference |
|---|---|---|---|
| | | mathematically this is equal to the inverse of the variance. This method assumes that all of the trials have measured the outcome on the same scale. | |
| Meta-analysis | — | The use of statistical techniques in a systematic review to integrate the results of included studies. Sometimes misused as a synonym for systematic reviews, where the review includes a meta-analysis. | — |
| Montgomery–Asberg Depression Rating Scale | MADRS | Questionnaire that rates the severity of depression. | Montgomery SA and Asberg M. (1979) A new depression scale designed to be sensitive to change. *B J Psychiatry* **134**: 382–389. |
| Non-controlled studies | — | Observations made on individuals, usually receiving the same intervention, before and after an intervention but with no control group. | http://handbook.cochrane.org/ |
| Noradrenergic and specific serotonergic antidepressants | NaSSA | A class of antidepressants. They antagonise the α2-adrenergic receptor and certain serotonin receptors. | |
| Other Chinese medicine therapies | — | Other Chinese medicine therapies include all traditional therapies except Chinese herbal medicine and acupuncture, such as, *tai chi* 太极, *qigong* 气功, *tuina* 推拿 and cupping. | |
| PubMed | PubMed | Bibliographic database. | http://www.ncbi.nlm.nih.gov/pubmed |
| Randomised controlled trial | RCT | Clinical trial that uses a random method to allocate participants to treatment and control groups. | — |
| Rating Scale for Side Effects–Asberg | SERS | Questionnaire to assess the side effects of antidepressants. | |
| Risk of bias | — | Assessment of clinical trials to indicate if the results may overestimate or underestimate the true effect because of bias in study design or reporting. | http://handbook.cochrane.org/ |

(*Continued*)

## (*Continued*)

| Terms | Acronym | Definition | Reference |
|---|---|---|---|
| Risk ratio (relative risk) | RR | The ratio of risks in two groups. In intervention studies, it is the ratio of the risk in the intervention group to the risk in the control group. A risk ratio of one indicates no difference between comparison groups. For undesirable outcomes, a risk ratio that is less than one indicates that the intervention was effective in reducing the risk of that outcome. | http://handbook.cochrane.org/ |
| Standardised mean difference | SMD | In meta-analysis: A method used to combine results for continuous scales which measure the same outcome, but measure it in different ways (e.g. with different scales). The results of studies are standardised to a uniform scale to allow data to be combined. | http://handbook.cochrane.org/ |
| Selective serotonin reuptake inhibitors | SSRI | SSRIs are a class of antidepressants used block the reuptake of serotonin in the brain. | |
| Serotonin norepinephrine reuptake inhibitors | SNRI | SNRIs are a class of antidepressants. Used to inhibit the reuptake of serotonin and norepinephrine. | |
| Summary of findings | — | Presentation of results and rating the quality of evidence based on the GRADE approach. | http://www.gradeworkinggroup.org/ |
| Transcutaneous electrical nerve stimulation | TENS | Application of transdermal electrical current to acupuncture points via conducting pads | — |
| Treatment Emergent Symptom Scale | TESS | Used to assess adverse events of treatments. The TESS reviews all body systems and documents the presence, absence, and intensity of 28 symptoms. | National Institute of Mental Health. (1985) TESS (Treatment Emergent Symptom Scale-Write-in). *Psychopharmacol Bull* **21**: 1069–1072. |
| Tricyclic antidepressants | TCA | A class of antidepressants that increase the levels of norepinephrine and serotonin. | |
| *Tuina* 推拿 | — | Chinese massage: Rubbing, kneading, or percussion of the soft tissues and joints of the body with the hands, usually performed by one person on another, esp. to relieve tension or pain. | WHO International Standard Terminologies of Traditional Medicine in the Western Pacific Region. World Health Organisation; 2007. |

*(Continued)*

| Terms | Acronym | Definition | Reference |
|---|---|---|---|
| Wangfang database | Wanfang | Chinese language bibliographic database. | www.wanfangdata.com |
| World Health Organisation | WHO | WHO is the directing and coordinating authority for health within the United Nations system. It is responsible for providing leadership on global health matters, shaping the health research agenda, setting norms and standards, articulating evidence-based policy options, providing technical support to countries and monitoring and assessing health trends. | http://www.who.int/about/en/ |
| World Health Organisation Quality of Life Scale Brief Version | WHOQOL-BREF | A quality of life assessment that includes physical, psychological, social relationships, and environmental domains. | Harper H, Power M and Group TW. (1998) Development of the World Health Organization WHOQOL-BREF quality of life assessment. *Psychol Med* **28**: 551–558. |
| Years lived with disability | YLD | YLDs are a measurement of the burden of disease. Calculated by multiplying the prevalence of a disorder by the short- or long-term loss of health associated with that disability. | https://www.nimh.nih.gov/health/statistics/disability/what-are-ylds.shtml |
| *Zhong Hua Yi Dian* 中华医典 | ZHYD | The Zhong Hua Yi Dian (ZHYD) "Encyclopaedia of Traditional Chinese Medicine" is a comprehensive series of electronic books on compact disk. The collection was put together by the Hunan electronic and audio-visual publishing house. It is the largest collection of Chinese electronic books and includes the major Chinese ancient works, many of which are from rare manuscripts and are the only existing copies. These books cover the period from ancient times up to the period of the Republic of China (1911–1948). | Hu R. (ed.) (2000) *Zhong Hua Yi Dian [Encyclopaedia of Traditional Chinese Medicine]*. 4th ed. Hunan Electronic and Audio-Visual Publishing House, Chengsha. |
| Zung Self-rating Depression Scale | SDS | Questionnaire that rates the severity of depression. | Zung WW. (1965) A self-rating depression scale. *Arch Gen Psychiatry* **12**: 63–70. |

# Index

acupuncture, 31, 46, 47, 133–154, 178

adverse events, 56, 57, 90, 144, 161, 166, 182

*An shen ding zhi tang* 安神定志汤, 74, 94, 175, 176

antidepressant, 1, 5, 6, 10–15

*Bai shao* 白芍, 117, 119, 127, 183

BL15 *Xinshu* 心腧, 47, 50

blood, 22, 23, 175, 177

*Chai hu* 柴胡, 44, 96, 101, 102, 118–119, 183

*Chai hu shu gan san* 柴胡疏肝散, 24, 72, 74, 93, 102–104, 175, 177

Chinese herbal medicine, 24, 41, 117, 173

combination therapies, 163–169

cupping, 159, 161, 168, 180–181

depressed mood, 1, 7, 8

diet therapy, 33, 180

*Di huang* 地黄, 117, 125

Edinburgh Postnatal Depression Scale (EPDS), 59, 87

electro-acupuncture, 133, 144, 178

fatigue, 1, 4, 7, 26, 31, 95, 150

fluoxetine, 13, 80, 81, 85, 86, 141, 143, 161, 168

*Fu ling* 茯苓, 44, 50

*Gan cao* 甘草, 50, 96, 101, 102, 121

*Gan mai da zao tang* 甘麦大枣汤, 31, 41–43, 50

GRADE, 62, 63, 89, 150

*Gui pi tang/wan* 归脾汤/丸, 30, 42, 103

GV20 *Baihui* 百会, 137, 144, 148, 150, 153

Hamilton Rating Scale for Depression (HRSD), 56, 77–86, 138–142, 145–147, 151, 152

heart, 21–25, 28–33, 40, 41

HT7 *Shenmen* 神门, 31, 137, 150, 153

kidney, 21–25, 29, 30

LI4 *Hegu* 合谷, 31, 32

liver, 21–29, 32, 33

Liver *qi* stagnation, 22, 24, 173, 177, 178, 180, 183

LR3 *Taichong* 太冲, 31, 137, 150, 153, 180

major depressive disorder, 1, 9
menopausal depression, 77, 79, 81, 84, 85, 104–106
Montgomery–Asberg Depression Rating Scale (MADRS), 58, 87, 143, 174
moxibustion, 45–47, 163, 168, 169

neurotransmitter, 6, 120, 123
non-controlled studies, 53–55
non-randomised controlled trials, 53, 55

PC6 *Neiguan* 内关, 47, 50, 138, 144, 150, 153, 179, 180
phlegm, 22–27, 41, 45, 46, 49
postpartum depression, 70, 77, 79, 81, 84, 85, 87, 104–106, 140–142
psychotherapy, 9, 11, 14, 175

*Qigong* 气功, 165, 167, 169

randomised controlled trials, 53
*Ren shen* 人参, 30, 42–44, 50
risk of bias, 60–63

Selective serotonin reuptake inhibitors (SSRI), 13, 77, 79, 80–84, 140–142, 146

*Shen* 神, 22
SP6 *Sanyinjiao* 三阴交, 32, 137, 150, 153, 180, 184
spleen, 21–27, 30–33
suicide, 3, 7–10
systematic review, 53–55, 62

*Taichi* 太极, 165, 167, 169
Treatment Emergent Symptom Scale (TESS), 56, 91, 92, 94, 97, 144, 151
*tuina* 推拿, 159, 161

unipolar depression, 1, 7

*Xiao yao san* 逍遥散, 46, 69, 73, 92, 126, 175, 177

*Yintang* (EX-HN3) 印堂, 137, 150, 179
*Yuan zhi* 远志, 117, 122
*Yu bing* 郁病, 21, 22

Zung Self-rating Depression Scale (SDS), 58, 86, 101, 143, 145, 147, 148

# Evidence-based Clinical Chinese Medicine

Print ISSN: 2529-7562
Online ISSN: 2529-7554

Series Co Editors-in-Chief

**Charlie Changli Xue** *(RMIT University, Australia)*
**Chuanjian Lu** *(Guangdong Provincial Hospital of Chinese Medicine, China)*

---

Published

Vol. 1    *Chronic Obstructive Pulmonary Disease*
          by Charlie Changli Xue and Chuanjian Lu

Vol. 2    *Psoriasis Vulgaris*
          Lead Authors: Claire Shuiqing Zhang and Jingjie Yu

Vol. 3    *Chronic Urticaria*
          Lead Authors: Meaghan Coyle and Jingjie Yu

Vol. 4    *Adult Asthma*
          Lead Authors: Johannah Shergis and Lei Wu

Vol. 5    *Allergic Rhinitis*
          Lead Authors: Claire Shuiqing Zhang and Qiulan Luo

Vol. 6    *Herpes Zoster and Post-herpetic Neuralgia*
          Lead Authors: Meaghan Coyle and Haiying Liang

Vol. 7    *Insomnia*
          Lead Authors: Johannah Shergis and Xiaojia Ni

Vol. 8    *Alzheimer's Disease*
          Lead Authors: Brian H May and Mei Feng

Vol. 9    *Vascular Dementia*
          Lead Authors: Brian H May and Mei Feng

Vol. 10   *Diabetic Kidney Disease*
          Lead Authors: Johannah Shergis and Lihong Yang

Vol. 11   *Acne Vulgaris*
          Lead Authors: Meaghan Coyle and Haiying Liang

More information on this series can also be found at https://www.worldscientific.com/series/ebccm

Vol. 12  *Post-Stroke Shoulder Complications*
         Lead Authors: Claire Shuiqing Zhang and Shaonan Liu

Vol. 14  *Unipolar Depression*
         Lead Authors: Yuan Ming Di and Lingling Yang

Vol. 16  *Atopic Dermatitis*
         Lead Authors: Meaghan Coyle and Junfeng Liu

Forthcoming

Vol. 13  *Post-Stroke Spasticity*
         Lead Authors: Claire Shuiqing Zhang and Shaonan Liu

Vol. 15  *Chronic Heart Failure*
         Lead Authors: Claire Shuiqing Zhang and Liuling Ma

Vol. 17  *Colorectal Cancer*
         Lead Authors: Brian H May and Yihong Liu